Truly Scrumptious Baby

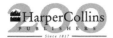

Thorsons
An imprint of HarperCollins*Publishers*
1 London Bridge Street
London SE1 9GF

www.harpercollins.co.uk

First published by Thorsons 2017

10 9 8 7 6 5 4 3 2 1

A catalogue record of this book is available from the British Library

ISBN 978-0-00-817256-5

Printed and bound in Slovenia

MIX
Paper from
responsible sources
FSC™ C007454

This book is produced from independently certified FSC paper to ensure responsible forest management.
For more information visit: www.harpercollins.co.uk/green

While the author has made every effort to ensure that the information contained in this book reflects NHS guidelines at the time of publication, medical knowledge is constantly changing and the application of it to particular circumstances depends on many factors. This book is intended as a reference volume only, not as a medical manual. The information given here is designed to help you make informed decisions about you and your baby, and it should be used to supplement rather than replace the advice of your doctor or other trained health professionals. Therefore it is recommended that a qualified medical specialist is always consulted for advice.

The nutrition and health claims made in this book have all been checked by a registered food nutritionist. All nutrition claims relating to ingredients themselves have been checked to ensure that they contain levels of macro or micronutrients that warrant a EU-registered nutrition claim. Any other health claims made have been researched and do not state fact but indicate that this is what research suggests. Recommendations throughout the book are based on UK guidelines. Once a child has reached a suitable age, all recipes should be eaten in the context of a healthy, balanced diet. The author and publishers cannot be held responsible for any errors and omissions that may be found in the text, or any actions that may be taken by a reader as a result of any reliance on the information contained in the text.

Mumsnet Rated: 46 Mumsnet testers reviewed a manuscript of this book in June 2017 – 89% would recommend *Truly Scrumptious Baby* and 81% would buy another book by Holly Willoughby.

HOLLY WILLOUGHBY

WITH KELLY WILLOUGHBY

Truly Scrumptious Baby

Thorsons

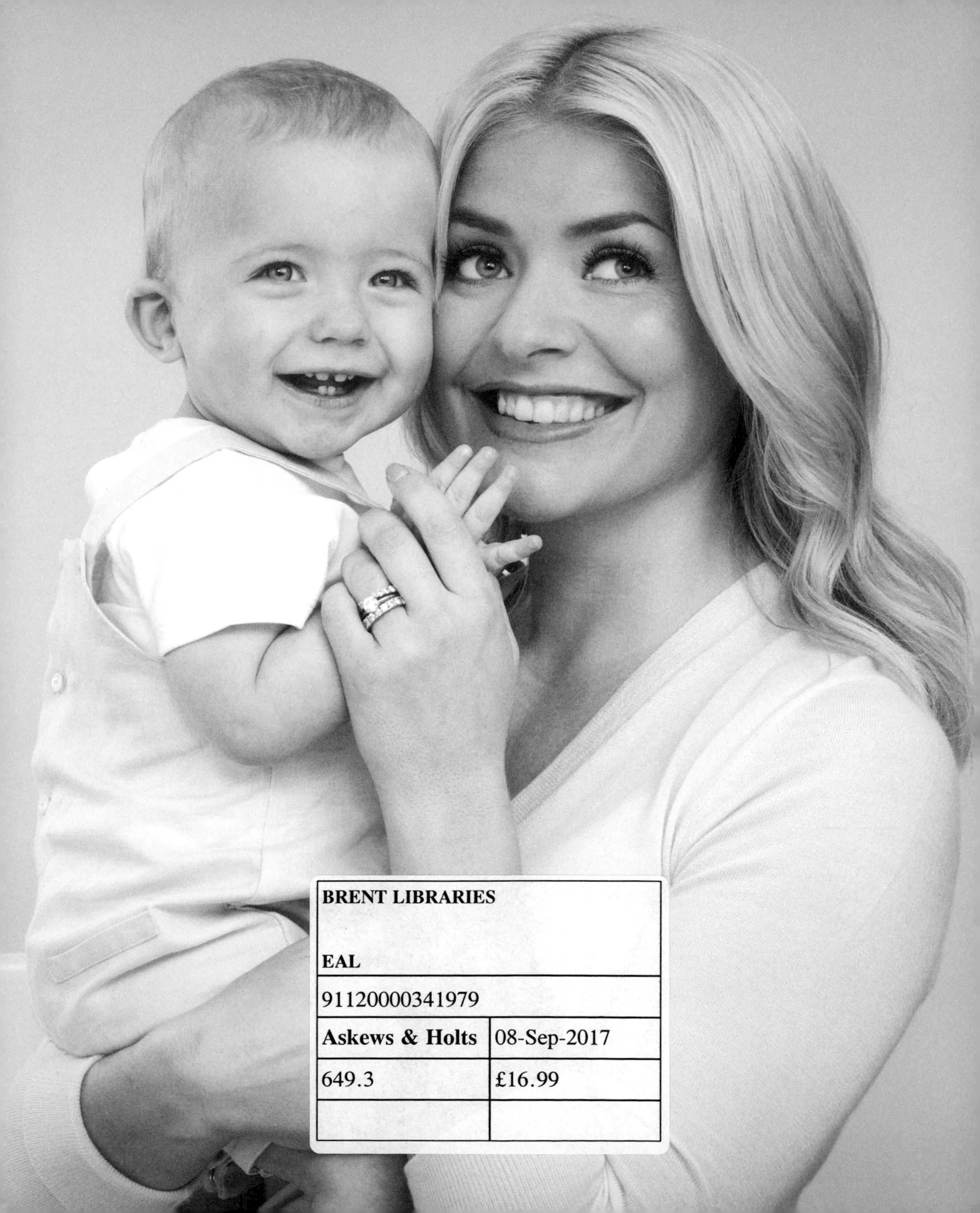

CONTENTS

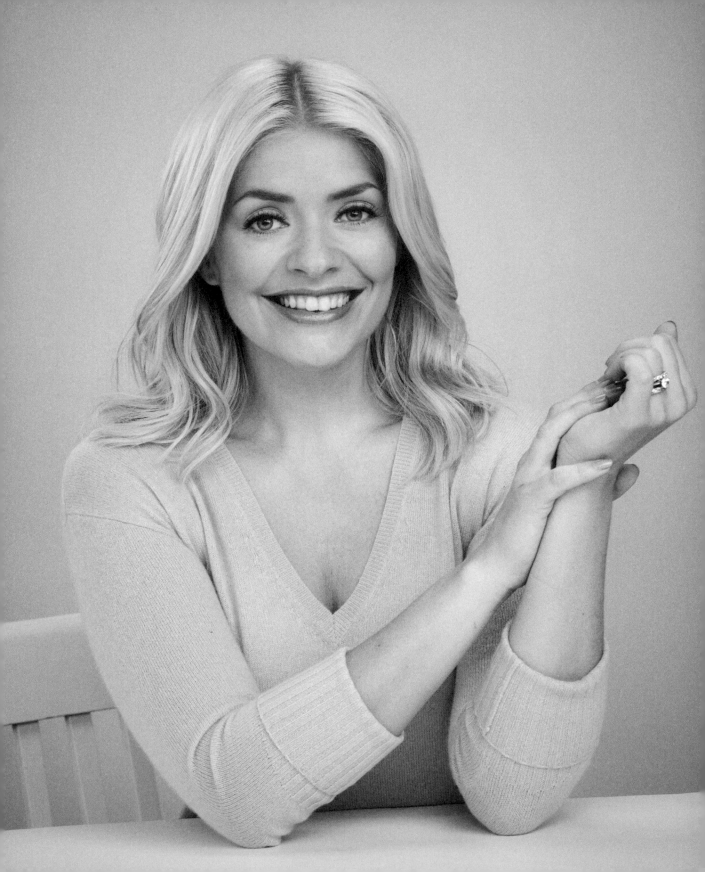

Hello again!

So here we are. Over the past six or so months, you and your baby have finally mastered the milk feed, and whether you've gone for breast or formula, all your hard work is plain to see in your baby's growing weight on the scales. Whether you've found the whole experience a doddle or a struggle, you've done it, and the results are squidgeable! But in this ever-evolving world of baby, it's time for change. It's time for the next exciting step: to introduce your little bundle to the colourful, flavourful and wonderful world of food – something that may well be met with mixed emotions!

You might fall into the camp of mothers who have exclusively breastfed since day one and loved every nursing moment, hence the thought of having to give up some of these feeds to foreign food matter is a bit threatening. You might be one of those mothers who loves the ease of milk (whether breast or bottle) and so the thought of having to add the preparation of food to your already busy routine is simply horrifying. Or you might be the sort of mum who's hated the whole milk-only phase and can't wait to start cramming the freezer with ice cubes of liquidized carrot. Whichever category you fall into, the simple truth is that the time has come and you have to embrace the solid, for the good of your baby and her development.

It's true that the thought of weaning can make even the most self-assured of mothers feel daunted. Not least because, as usual, there are decisions to be made. Do you go down the traditional route of spoon-feeding your little one lump-free purées, or do you investigate the newer 'baby-led weaning' approach and let your baby feed herself from the moment solid food first touches her lips? As with everything, there are no right or wrong answers. I'm just here to try to arm you with options for making your own informed choices about what will work best for you, your baby and indeed the rest of your family.

When I started this project, I reflected on all those things I had wanted to know as a parent when I embarked on weaning for the first time: when to start, for example, and how to know if my baby was ready. I wanted to know how to prepare myself for the daunting task ahead, what equipment to buy and how to move from one stage to the next. I wanted simple, easy-to-follow recipes, made with economical ingredients that pack a nutritional punch. I certainly didn't want to waste money on expensive weaning gadgets, or spend lots of time in the kitchen on fiddly recipes that left me with a ton of washing-up. To top it all, I wanted to know exactly what challenges I might face and how to manage them.

So, in this book, I hope to provide you with all this information, and more. In my experience, the weaning process can be tricky to master and varies for every baby – there will be changes to your routine and potentially some frustrating moments. But even when there's more food on the floor than in your baby's tummy, one thing I can guarantee if you follow the recipes in this book is that you'll be catering to her nutritional needs at each stage of the weaning process. Each recipe has been developed to ensure that your little one gets the correct balance of nutrients every step of the way. Minimum fuss, maximum benefit is my motto. And I hope this will allow you to have a bit of fun with food, to make mealtimes appealing for your little one – without losing your sanity in the process!

For my part, I absolutely loved the experience of taking all of mine through the various weaning stages. I can remember each of their faces when that first spoonful of baby rice touched their lips. So best of luck, fellow feeders! And try not to stress. Remember the mantra that every baby is unique and your baby will get there in the end. How many adults do you know who are still living on a diet of puréed fruit?!

Come on – we can do this!

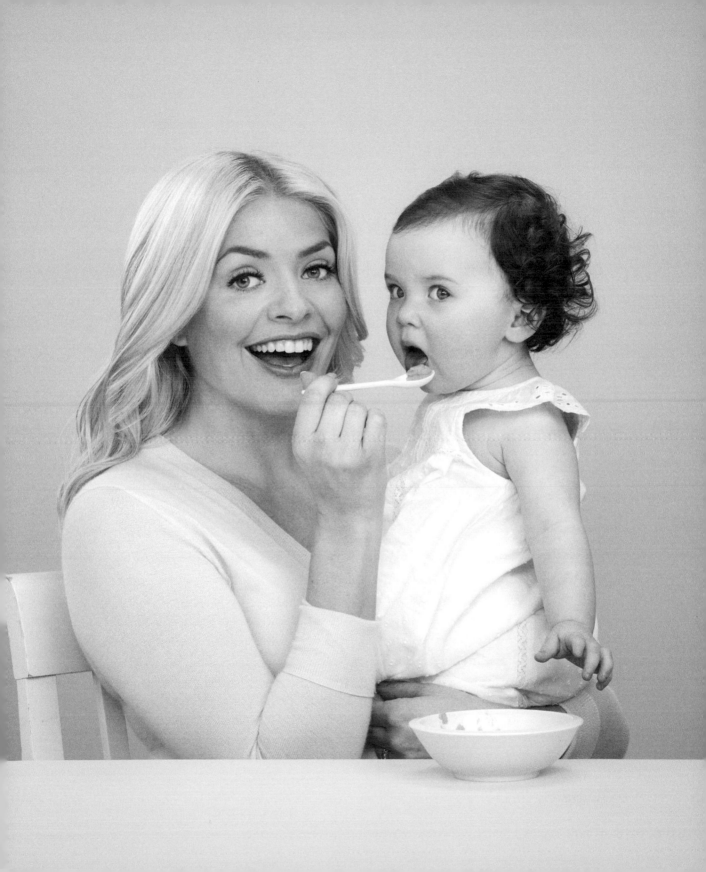

INTRODUCTION TO FEEDING

THE IMPORTANCE OF GOOD NUTRITION FROM THE WORD GO

As parents, I think we have a responsibility to give our children the best possible dietary start in life. Right from the very first spoonful of purée, it's never too early to instil healthy eating habits. Indeed, the more key nutrients your baby consumes, the better equipped he'll be for all the growth spurts to come. Our diet affects our immune system, our metabolism and our cognitive function, and it has a measurable effect on our physical development. What we eat has a direct impact on energy levels, sleep, hair, skin and oral health – and that's just for starters. It doesn't take long before the quality of our diet, at whatever age, begins to show in our well-being. It's amazing, really, how something we are completely in control of, in terms of the choices we make, can affect us so tangibly.

Encouraging your child to have a positive relationship with food extends beyond what he's eating, though. Helping him to develop a healthy attitude towards mealtimes is essential for when he's older, and there are a few simple things you can do to encourage this when weaning, such as not using food as a bribe (tempting though this may be!). You'll find more about this on pages 33–4.

MOVING FROM MILK TO SOLIDS

In the first few months of your baby's life, what to feed him has never been an issue. Whether breast or formula, milk has been his sole form of nourishment, providing him with complete nutrition. And, according to NHS guidelines, milk should remain your baby's sole source of nutrition until six months of age. He simply isn't ready physiologically to take in solid food before four months, in fact, and while you might offer simple purées alongside his usual milk from four months, there is no advantage in doing so. After six months, whether in the form of purées or mashed meals or finger foods, your baby can start to take in nutrients from solid food. For the first few months of weaning, milk is still king when it comes to nutrition, however, as he will only really be exploring and playing with food; it won't be sustaining him yet. Then, as he consumes more than he drops, and the more balanced his diet of solid foods becomes, food will gradually over time become more dominant and milk less so. But when it comes to taking that first step from milk to solids, where do you begin?

WHERE TO START?

The world of solids can be a minefield, especially with so much conflicting advice out there.

'Babies and children need fats' – but not too many of the bad ones.
'Sugar is the route of all evil' – but it's in everything!
'Carbs are great for energy' – but too many of the wrong ones make you sluggish.

Where do you even start without signing up for a degree in nutrition? That's how it can seem to a new parent. In reality, it's not so complicated, however. It's all about tapping into the basics of what you already know about eating healthily to help you make the right food choices for your baby. If someone offers you an apple or a chocolate biscuit and asks you to pick the healthy option, it's a no-brainer. But if they offered you two bowls of mashed potato, which looked identical but contained different ingredients, which would you choose? You would have no idea unless you'd cooked it yourself and knew what was in it – and that's the bottom line. When it comes to eating healthily, a homemade dish gives you the control to make the right choices for your baby. 'But that's obvious!' I hear you cry. 'And I just don't have time to start mashing potato, when the kids are hollering for their dinner!' In today's busy world, is it any wonder that we are drawn to the convenience of pre-packed supermarket mashed potato? And no one can blame us for that. But when you make your own, you know it's not packed full of salt and additives – you have complete control. That said, not all supermarket convenience foods need to be avoided. I'm all for things like frozen vegetables and pre-chopped onions or other pre-prepared veggies if they make home cooking that little bit speedier when time is short.

If you strip everything back and think about what we take from food, it's easy to understand why we need a balanced diet. Different food groups contain different nutrients, so we need to eat a good cross-section in order to obtain all the necessary goodness to perform at our best.

FOOD GROUPS AND GETTING THE BALANCE RIGHT

Fruits and vegetables

(e.g. apples, bananas, oranges, carrots and tomatoes) Fruits and vegetables contain vitamins and minerals that keep our bodies healthy and help us fight illness.

Starchy carbohydrates

(e.g. bread, rice, potatoes and pasta) These give us energy.

Protein

(e.g. meat, fish, eggs, nuts, legumes and tofu) Protein helps our bodies to grow and repair.

Dairy

(e.g. milk, cheese, yoghurt and alternatives) Dairy contains calcium and vitamin D, which help to keep our bones and teeth healthy and strong.

Fats and sugary foods

(e.g. butter, oil and sweets) We need a small amount of fat to help us to grow and to protect our organs. Too much fat and sugar can be very bad for your health.

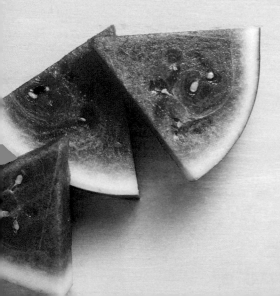

A baby's diet varies slightly from an adult's in terms of the weighting between each of these food groups. For example, where an adult's diet should be high in fibre and lower in fat, babies need more fat but less fibre as it's very filling. Crucially, babies also need a wide selection of vitamins and minerals to support healthy development. Largely these are found naturally in the foods we eat, although some parents choose to bolster their baby's intake of these nutrients with supplements (see page 16); others are recommended to all children in the UK.

avocado

Avocado is a source of vitamin E, which helps to **protect our cells** (the tiny building blocks of our body) against damage so we can stay healthy and strong.

banana

Bananas are a source of a mineral called potassium. Our **muscles need potassium in order to work** and contract properly.

broccoli

Broccoli is a source of vitamin C, folic acid, potassium and fibre. Potassium helps our nervous system to keep working efficiently.

butternut squash

Squash is a source of vitamins A, E and C. **Vitamin E helps protect our cells** against damage.

carrot

Carrots are a great source of beta carotene, which our body converts to vitamin A. **Vitamin A helps us to be able to see properly.** Without enough vitamin A we wouldn't be able to see very well in the dark.

courgette

Courgettes are a source of potassium. Potassium keeps our muscles working efficiently.

green bean

Grean beans are a great source of a mineral called **magnesium, which helps us to build muscle** so we can become strong and healthy.

peach

Peaches are a good source of **vitamin C, which helps to keep our bones, teeth and skin healthy.**

papaya

Papayas are one of the fruits with the highest vitamin C content. They are also a good source of vitamin A and fibre.

pea

Peas are a source of thiamin (vitamin B1), vitamin C, folic acid and fibre. **Vitamin C helps to keep our immune system healthy and protects our cells against damage.**

sweet potato

Sweet potato is a source of vitamins A, E and C, as well as potassium and copper. **Copper aids our metabolism and is vital for the production of red and white blood cells.**

Here are some of the key vitamins and minerals babies need at various stages of their development, and what they're needed for. When weaning my little ones, I found it incredibly helpful to know a bit about the nutritional content of the ingredients I was using.

Vitamin A

Vitamin A (also known as retinol) is important for keeping **eyes and skin healthy**. There are two forms of vitamin A: retinol, found in animal sources, and beta-carotene, found in plant sources, which are converted to vitamin A in the body. Vitamin A aids the **immune system**, so it's vital for keeping little bodies healthy and warding off illness, and it's also important for **healthy vision**. It's found in lots of foods that can be introduced from six months, including eggs, cheese, yoghurt, carrot, butternut squash, sweet potato, kale, spinach, apricot and mango. Liver and liver products are also very high in vitamin A and can be given to children once a week from 12 months.

Vitamin C

Vitamin C is really important to our immune system. It helps **protect our cells** from stress and aids iron absorption. It also contributes to **healthy teeth and skin**, and it helps with **psychological function** and the **reduction of tiredness** and fatigue. Vitamin C is found in a wide range of foods, all of which may be introduced from six months onwards, including especially tomatoes, peppers, broccoli, potatoes, cauliflower, cabbage, peaches, papaya, blueberries, raspberries, strawberries, oranges and kiwi fruit.

Vitamin D

Vitamin D is crucial for **healthy bones, teeth and muscles**. It helps our bodies absorb calcium, which in turn promotes bone growth and strength. Most vitamin D is obtained from exposure to sunlight. Just make sure your little ones have plenty of UV protection on if they're out enjoying the sunshine! Vitamin D is also found in eggs, oily fish (as long as it's not smoked) and red meat, which can be given to babies from six months, and liver and liver products, which can be given to children once a week from 12 months (this is due to the very high vitamin A content of liver).

Calcium

Calcium is one of the main minerals for building **strong bones** and **healthy teeth**. It's important to give your little one's body strong foundations so that it will support him well throughout life. Calcium works with vitamin D to help children's bones grow and develop healthily. It's also important for a host of bodily functions including **digestion, muscle contraction and metabolism**.

Calcium is found in yoghurt, cheese, broccoli and leafy green vegetables. It's also found in cow's milk, which can be included in meals from six months but not given as a main milk feed to babies under a year.

Iron

Iron is a must for babies. It plays a vital role in **cognitive development** in children and therefore can affect intellectual performance. It also helps to make haemoglobin, found in red blood cells – the little fellas that carry oxygen around the blood. If you don't have enough iron, you can feel really tired and dizzy. Up to six months in age, babies get all the iron they need from breast milk or formula, so when you start to reduce that source, you need to introduce iron-rich foods. These include most dark leafy greens, red meat, ground nuts and pulses. And also liver and liver products, which you can give to children once a week from 12 months (this is due to the very high vitamin A content of liver).

Zinc

Zinc is needed for the functioning of every organ in the body. It plays a major role in the **metabolism** of macronutrients and **wound healing**, and it helps to keep our **hair, nails and skin healthy**. It's found in foods such as eggs, poultry, beans, lentils, ground nuts, sesame seeds and tofu. And also liver and liver products, which can be given to children once a week from 12 months (this is due to the very high vitamin A content of liver).

SUPPLEMENTS

Even if you're mindful of nutrition and aware of how to source all the crucial vitamins and minerals your baby needs from different types of food, it's still advisable to boost his diet with a few supplements. According to NHS guidelines, children between six months and five years will benefit from daily supplements of vitamins A, C and D. Vitamin D is particularly important and the NHS advice suggests that breastfed babies should receive supplements containing 8.5 to 10mcg of vitamin D from birth. For formula-fed babies, it isn't necessary until they're having less than 500ml/18fl oz of infant formula a day. Between the ages of one and four, children should be given a daily supplement of 10mcg of vitamin D.

Your health visitor can give advice on where to buy vitamin drops and who is eligible to receive them free of charge. It's crucial to remember, though, that overdoing the vitamins can be harmful, so make sure you keep to the recommended daily doses. (Foods that contain too much of a particular vitamin should be avoided in your baby's first year too – see pages 18–20.)

ALLERGIES

I know that many new parents are concerned about allergies. Common allergy trigger foods include nuts and seeds; cow's milk; fish and shellfish; wheat and eggs. Your baby could have a higher risk if you have a significant family history of food allergies or of atopic illnesses such as eczema, asthma and hay fever. If you think this genetic disposition applies to you, I would definitely advise having a discussion with your GP about how carefully to tread when beginning the weaning process with your little one with regards to introducing known allergens, especially peanuts, if there is a known allergy to other nuts or a family history of peanut allergy. It won't necessarily follow that your baby will be allergic to these foods, but it is worth being extra careful. At six months, not before, you should introduce allergens slowly and one at a time until you are happy there's no kind of reaction. On the bright side breastfeeding can help reduce the risk of allergies and babies often grow out of an allergy, although a peanut allergy is usually for life. Try to avoid experimenting by cutting out whole food groups unless advised by a medical professional such as a dietician.

Vegetarian

I know many vegetarians who have successfully weaned their babies on a vegetarian diet. There are just a few things you need to keep in mind if you're planning to do so. A vegetarian diet is often higher in fibre and contains less energy-dense foods. This means that young children may not have the appetite to eat enough to provide all the nutrients they need and so a little bit more planning can be required. To keep everything in check nutritionally, focus on giving your baby lots of variety, so things like dark green vegetables (e.g. Blueberry, Apple and Spinach purée – see page 70), beans and lentils (e.g. Squash and Red Lentil purée – see page 72) dairy and eggs (e.g. Tomato Quinoa Bowl – see page 90) and some dried fruit, too, such as apricots, figs and dates. It's also helpful to know that vitamin C helps the body to absorb iron, so try to regularly include some fruit or veggies, in which it's found in abundance.

Vegan

Weaning a baby on a vegan diet does require a little more planning but many of the points above still stand, and it is possible for a baby to get all the nutrients he needs from a balanced and varied diet. Energy density of food can be a concern as vegan food is often high in fibre but not very energy dense. Foods such as hummus, tahini, bananas, nut or seed butters (see page 280) dried fruit, nutritional yeast and fortified (unsweetened) milk make great additions but it does all come back to balance and variety. It is worth being aware of the key micronutrients mentioned on page 15 as well as vitamin B12 and iodine, and perhaps considering the supplements mentioned on page 16, as well as seeking advice from a qualified dietician.

INTRODUCING FOODS GRADUALLY

According to NHS guidelines, there are some foods that should be avoided altogether for the first year of life for different reasons.

FOODS TO AVOID IN THE FIRST YEAR

Cow's milk as a main milk feed

While cow's milk can be given during weaning as part of a meal, it shouldn't take the place of your baby's usual milk during the first year as it doesn't contain all the essential nutrients your baby needs for this important stage of development and for protection against illness. So stick to breast milk or formula for the first year. They contain all the essential nutrients your baby needs to grow properly. Should you choose to stop breast feeding, there is no advantage to moving to follow-on milks. From 12 months infants, provided they are healthy, should be eating a wide variety of foods and this will be their main source of nutrients. They should also be drinking around 400ml/14fl oz of whole animal milk (either cow, goat or sheep's milk), or a suitable substitute.

Raw eggs and other uncooked foods

You can give your baby eggs, but ensure that both the white and yolk are cooked solid. Don't forget, too, that some pre-packed foods contain raw eggs, so do read any labels carefully to avoid these. In general, any unpasteurized food should be avoided during the first year as it can cause food poisoning. Meat and fish should always be well cooked.

Low-fat foods

Low-fat products should be avoided during the first year as they will probably not be energy dense enough for your baby's nutritional needs.

Fibrous foods

Foods that are too fibrous and limit the absorption of some minerals, such as bran-based cereals and breads, should be avoided during the first year. High-fibre foods, such as whole grains, should only be given in small quantities.

Whole nuts and seeds and other hard foods

The latest NHS advice is to avoid giving a baby under five any whole nuts to avoid choking. It's also best to avoid giving young children chunks of hard food, such as apple or cheese, as these are also a potential choking hazard. Once your baby is six months old and you are sure there is no immediate family history of food allergies, or eczema, asthma or hay fever, then you can introduce some ground nuts or nut products like peanut butter into your baby's diet, one by one, but take medical advice if you're unsure.

Shellfish and certain other fish

The super omega-3 fats found in fish are very beneficial to health. But be wary of some fish. Shark, marlin and swordfish contain high traces of mercury, which can damage an immature nervous system, so avoid those completely. And shellfish carry a higher risk of food poisoning, so it's best to steer clear of those, too, for the first year. There are plenty of other, safer fish options to try for the moment – just make sure to remove any bones!

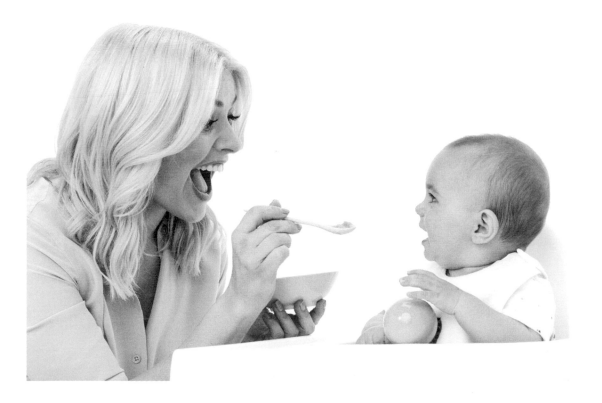

Liver and liver products

Liver and liver products such as liver pâté should not be given during the first year as they contain high levels of vitamin A, which can be harmful to your baby. Once your baby is 12 months old you can give them up to once a week.

Early weaning

If parents choose to introduce food before six months, then they should also exclude wheat and gluten in cereal foods such as bread and pasta, as well as eggs, nuts, seeds, liver, fish, shellfish and cow's milk or other dairy foods.

FOODS TO AVOID IN THE FIRST YEAR AND BEYOND

Rice milk

Traces of arsenic have been found to exist naturally in rice milk. The official advice is not to give it to children under the age of five. If your child has a dairy intolerance, other milk alternatives are available after your child is a year old. Just be sure that whatever milk you give your little one is fortified with the relevant vitamins and minerals his growing body needs. And check that it is unsweetened and not rice based.

Salt

Too much salt is detrimental at any age, but particularly for babies and small children as their underdeveloped kidneys can't process an excess of salt. As a rule, the family chef should leave seasoning out of home-cooked meals. Adults can always add their own at the table. Be aware that there are some everyday store-cupboard ingredients that are very high in salt but which may not be immediately obvious, such as stock cubes, gravy granules and soy sauce. Supermarkets do low-salt, baby-friendly alternatives to a lot of these, so have a look. And have a go at making your own salt-free stock! (See pages 109–11.)

Processed foods

Meat products such as sausages, burgers and chicken nuggets are standard fare for family meals, but unless you get these foods direct from a reputable butcher and can be sure the meat content is high, you have no idea what's really in them. As with other processed foods, there is a high chance that they will be full of salt, sugar and a myriad other detrimental additives and food colourings. Where possible, steer clear!

Refined sugar and artificial sweeteners

Sugar seems to be the number-one enemy today and there's no doubt in my mind that it can spark a change in children's behaviour. An excess of sugar, whether in the form of 'natural' sugar or artificial sweeteners, is linked to obesity, diabetes and heart problems. There are two types of sugars: naturally occurring ones found in whole fruit, vegetables and milk-based products, and free sugars, which are added to things like honey, syrups and fruit juices. The naturally occurring sugars are a good source of vitamins, minerals and fibre for your little one but just remember that habits are formed at a young age – if you're feeding them lots of sugary things, they'll develop a sweet tooth. There's nothing wrong with a little chocolate now and again, but moderation is key! And make sure to watch out for drinks such as fruit juices and squashes, which often contain huge quantities of sugar.

Artificial sweeteners should be avoided altogether – partly because there's lots of contradictory evidence around them and partly because they're *extremely* sweet! They'll give your little one a taste for sugar and it's best to avoid this at all costs!

Honey

Honey can contain spores, which can lead to infant botulism. Although the disease is fairly rare, it can be fatal, so it's best to leave honey out of your baby's diet for the first year. And try to limit your child's consumption of it after that. Honey might seem like a natural, healthy sweetener, but it has the same effect as sugar.

Caffeine

Be mindful that caffeine isn't just in tea and coffee – it's found in chocolate and also in some drinks made with sugar substitutes, so be careful to limit those. Too much caffeine can cause hyperactivity in children – not to mention anxiety, tummy problems and lack of sleep. No child – or parent, for that matter – needs that!

GETTING READY TO START

STOCKING THE WEANING KITCHEN

There are only a handful of fresh ingredients that I'd advise getting when you're preparing to embark on weaning. Plain full-fat live yoghurt, butter, cream cheese and hard cheese are really useful and have a slightly longer shelf life, but other than that, I'd urge you NOT to go out and buy every ingredient under the sun. Your baby can't possibly consume loads of fresh fruit and veg before it goes off, so unless you have a big family who will pick up the consumption slack, don't go overboard initially. Think of it rather like that enormous list your best friend gave you when you were pregnant, with a million and one things you supposedly need to buy for your baby's arrival. Remember, when your little one finally arrived, how many of those items were completely unnecessary, or you didn't need them until a bit further down the line.

STORE-CUPBOARD BASICS

Dry ingredients, on the other hand, are really useful to have in your cupboards from the off. It makes planning meals and batch cooking so much easier. If you have the space in your kitchen, you can bulk-buy these because they'll definitely get used and it's so much more cost effective.

Rice, Dried pasta, Couscous, Quinoa, Rolled porridge oats, Dried lentils, Tinned tomatoes, Tinned sweetcorn, Tinned tuna and Tinned beans

FREEZER

A freezer is not a complete necessity – if you don't have one, it doesn't take too long to cook and whizz up fresh meals – but it really can make life a whole lot easier in the weaning kitchen. Having a freezer is a real bonus, especially when it comes to making batches of food for your baby, allowing you to store them safely in individual portions to defrost as and when she needs a meal. Where you can freeze a recipe in this book, it is labelled 'suitable for freezing', and this applies to

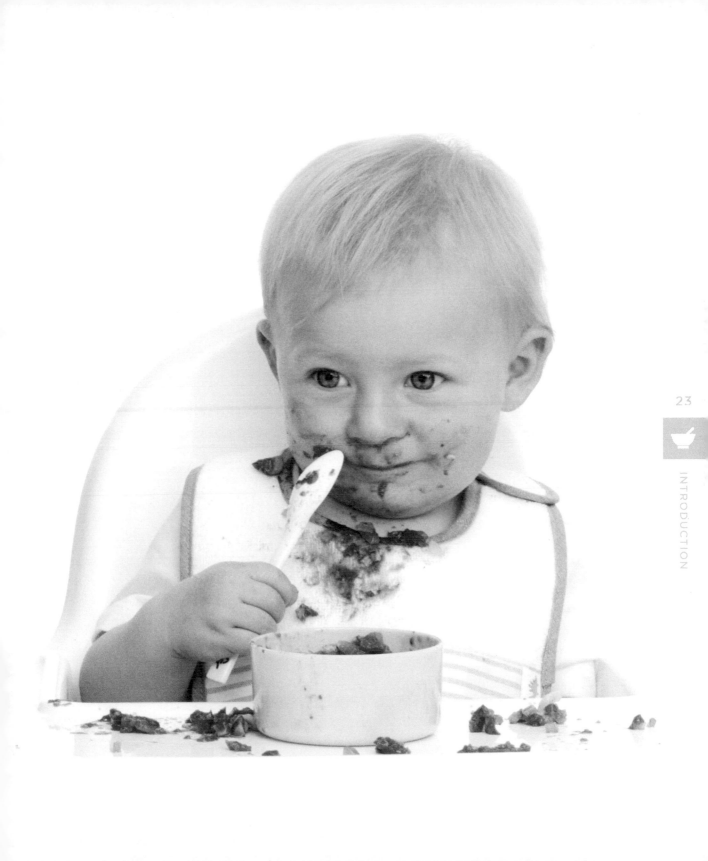

most of the purées and many of the other dishes that are suitable for serving to your baby with the rest of the family when she's a bit older.

Making space in the freezer

At some point – particularly if you are going down the classic purées route – you will need to set aside some freezer space for your lovingly made, single-ingredient purées. The key is to label everything. I keep a marker pen and a pack of labels on top of the freezer to mark up the date the food went in – and what it is! You'd be surprised how everything looks the same when frozen. I shouldn't out my mum, but she's served up an apple pie thinking it was a chicken pie on more than one occasion.

Silicone ice-cube trays/freezer bags

I've found that the best and most convenient way to store baby purées/mashes in an easily accessible way is to make up large batches of different individual vegetable and fruit purées, spoon them into ice-cube trays, cover with cling film and then freeze. As soon as it's frozen, pop the cubes of purée out into a freezer bag and add a label with the type of food and the date of freezing.

Once you've done a few different types of individual purée, and your baby is ready to move on from single-ingredient purées, you can defrost two or three and mix them together. By doing this, your baby is getting a variety of flavours and you're not having to start from scratch every day. One day she might have sweet potato and carrot. The next carrot and apple. If you count each cube as 20ml/¾fl oz in size, you can work out how many cubes to defrost according and there's minimal waste (compared with a shop-bought pouch that, once you open it, has to go in the bin if your baby can't finish it).

How long to keep things

If you do have a freezer and you're anything like me, it will be jam-packed full of foods you shove in and keep forgetting to use up! Anything containing meat can be stored in the freezer for a pretty long time and still be safe to eat, but the quality will deteriorate so it's best to eat it within 3–6 months. Remember, you should never refreeze raw meat or fish that has already been defrosted. You can safely refreeze meat that has been defrosted and cooked, and you can also do this with fish, though I find it changes the texture so I don't recommend it.

FOOD-STORAGE SAFETY

Once you've got going with weaning and stocked your freezer with batches of purée, there are a few more rules to follow to keep your little one safe from an upset tummy or worse.

Make sure you don't reheat any purées more than once after defrosting.

If you've made a purée and put it straight into the fridge, that's fine, but make sure it's in a pot with a lid or covered with cling film, and it absolutely has to be used within 24 hours from when you made it.

Frustrating though this might be, if you've only managed to dip the spoon into a bowl of purée a couple of times, and it's been in your baby's mouth – but she's not interested – don't keep it. Saliva transfer from your baby's mouth to the spoon, then to the purée, will have contaminated the food so it's just not safe to keep. Sorry!

As a precautionary measure during weaning, I don't recommend keeping or freezing leftover cooked rice as it's important to be incredibly careful when reheating it, due to the slight risk of food poisoning. Cooked rice should not be allowed to sit at room temperature for any length of time for the same reason.

GENERAL HYGIENE IN THE KITCHEN

You'll be used to keeping everything clean since the arrival of your little one, especially if you feel like you've spent more time with your sterilizer in the last six months than with friends and family! But, just in case, here's a quick checklist:

Wash hands and dry with a clean tea towel. If you use one you've had lying around the kitchen for ages, there's literally no point in having washed your hands in the first place.

Wipe down your kitchen work space with disinfectant every time you use it.

Make sure all weaning equipment has been washed in hot soapy water/put through the dishwasher/sterilized, though you don't have to sterilize anything other than bottles after six months.

COOKING EQUIPMENT

As with fresh ingredients, there is really no need to go mad when it comes to stocking up on cooking equipment. You'll find you most likely can get by on what you have already. I had one of those purée cooker gadgets to which you add food and water, push a button, and it steams and purées in about 15 minutes. It was great, and they've probably come on a lot since I bought mine, but considering how quickly your baby will move on from super-smooth purées, I think it's a lot of money to spend for the short amount of time you use it. Here are a few things that I wouldn't be without, though.

Food processor/blender

You'll need some sort of food processor or blender to make purées for your baby in the early months, though again, there's no need to spend a huge amount of money as this stage is relatively short, and you'll soon be on to mashing. That said, unless you're going to be making quite big batches of purée with a view to stocking up the freezer, a mini food processor or blender is the best size for the small amounts of each ingredient you're going to cook and whizz up. You can otherwise pick up a hand blender relatively cheaply and that will more than suffice for whizzing up small amounts. In the recipes, you'll find that I try to give different options wherever possible.

Saucepan/steamer

A basic saucepan with a lid is great for boiling vegetables and poaching fruit for purées – and that is how they have been cooked in the recipes here, with some of the cooking water then being used to thin purées in the early stages – but I'd highly recommend you invest in a steamer. This doesn't have to be an expensive stand-alone steaming gadget; just one of those little metal baskets that sit inside a lidded saucepan will suffice. Steaming is a good way to preserve certain nutrients, and the minimal cooking water will be easily absorbed into your meal, retaining more of the goodness of the ingredients.

Microwave

There's no doubt about it – a microwave is a wonderful modern convenience when it comes to speedy reheating or defrosting. It's a super-easy way to steam vegetables too. Just make sure that you are well versed in how your own microwave works, so that you know how to use it safely in terms of having it on the correct cook and defrost settings. If you're reheating food, be careful about 'hotspots'. Pause it and stir once or twice during cooking to make sure the heat is evenly dispersed. And, as with everything, make sure the temperature is just right before you offer it to your baby.

Potato masher

Once you've moved on from smooth purées, you'll need something to mash the cooked food so it retains more texture. Depending on how much you've made, a potato masher is handy, or just use the back of a fork!

FEEDING EQUIPMENT

I think the bottom line when it comes to purchasing anything baby related is to try making do without it and if you feel you absolutely can't, then pop out to buy or order it. The biggest budget-busting mistake all new parents make – and I'm no exception – is to rush out and buy everything on 'the list', thinking they'll fail without it, when every baby's needs are different and some just pass certain stages altogether and suddenly you're left with a load of gadgets that haven't even seen the light of day! But here are a few trusty basics that I couldn't have managed without.

Baby chair

You don't need to spend a fortune on a baby chair! In my experience, the more expensive they are and the more space age they look, the trickier they are to clean and the less supportive they are. There are plenty of chair options on the market, at a range of prices to suit your budget. Whatever you decide to go for, it must be supportive. If your baby is at the weaning stage, she should be strong enough to sit up straight and have good head control. The Bumbo-type seats are suitable for really early stages and some even come with detachable trays. If you are putting your baby straight into a high chair, make sure she's comfortable, well supported and strapped in. Ones with detachable trays have the advantage of flexibility, in that your child can either eat on her own or the chair can be pulled up to the table. If you're opting for a chair that either attaches to or pulls up to your own table, without a detachable tray, make sure it's safe. Chairs that can be clipped onto the table or fold up are especially good if you're short on space.

I used a Bumbo, followed by a Tripp Trapp high chair that pulled straight up to the table –with a baby harness for when my kids were really little. But that's just what worked for me, allowing me to sit and eat with them. The chair, which can be adjusted as your child gets bigger, was particularly handy when the second and third children came along as they could then eat with the older ones. It's no coincidence that Chester is my best eater. He's learned by example from watching the other two with their ever-maturing taste buds, and, at two years old, I can honestly say there's nothing that child won't eat. (Except mashed potato, that is. He hates mashed potato!)

It's quite a good idea to let your baby become acclimatized to her new high chair in the week running up to starting weaning. Giving her a weaning spoon to play with, along with a plastic bowl, plate or cup, while you eat your dinner, is a good way of introducing her to sitting down to a family meal and getting used to it before you add food to the party! Babies don't miss a trick. They'll be taking it all in, watching and learning, so by the time their turn comes, it won't feel so foreign.

Bowls and spoons

There are all sorts of brilliant feeding products on the market. You can now buy silicone bowls and spoons in heat-sensitive materials that change colour if the food's too hot, and I think that's a terrific idea. If I was going to go out again now and buy a set for a first baby, I think I would definitely go for the bowls with suckers that attach to the table so that they can't be knocked sideways! But any bowl that won't smash if it ends up on the floor is fine.

The only must with weaning spoons is that they need to be made from soft plastic or silicone. This is to protect your baby's gums as she eats. It's worth having a couple of spoons as babies often respond better to being fed if they are also holding a spoon and feel like they're doing it themselves. Giving them this sense of independence helps them develop their motor skills, too, and it won't be long before they're scooping up their own spoonfuls and accurately popping them into their mouths.

Sippy cup

From six months, you can encourage your baby to take a few sips of water from a spout beaker or 'sippy' alongside her new 'solid' meal. You can get ones with handles, to make it easier for little hands to control, and she'll love the feeling of independence that comes with this new experience. I would advise investing in a cup with a lid, but one that allows the water to flow freely rather than the non-spill type. This teaches your baby how to sip and drink properly, and it will stand her in good stead for when it's time to lose the lid and start drinking from an open cup with the sipping control they've unwittingly learned. Teaching your child how to use a straw early on is also a godsend. Once they master this, it makes things so much easier when you're out and about. Mine learned by watching me and Dan. I'd suck liquid through the straw and then let it go and blow a few bubbles. I know this sounds as though you'd be teaching your children bad habits, but it's enough to spark their interest and show them how to draw up liquid and watch how it moves up and down the straw. All of mine learned really quickly and it definitely helped with learning to sip and drink properly.

Bibs

When my babies were at the milk-only stage, I used those super-soft milk-feeding bibs with the padded ridge around the neck, which soaked up all the drips and leaks, helping to prevent rashes. But bibs for weaning are a totally different ball game. Essentially, you still want one to catch the excess – but this time you'll want one you can wipe clean, or you'll be spending a fortune on stain remover! You can get silicone ones with inbuilt trays. Inevitably they don't catch everything – but I've always been glad it's there.

Face cloth/muslin/wipes

You'll need something to wipe your baby down once they've finished eating. Just make sure it's something clean – and not the kitchen J-cloth! Equally, if you're using baby wipes, try them on your own face first. Some are fine to use on little hands, but quite scratchy on their sensitive faces and you won't know until you try it yourself. As a rule, try not to wipe your baby's face too much mid-feed, even if she is covered in goo. You risk aggravating and distracting her before she's full.

Sterilizer

You only need to sterilize your feeding equipment if you're weaning a baby under six months old. Any work-surface or microwave-bottle sterilizer will work. After that, it's fine to hand wash or put everything through the dishwasher.

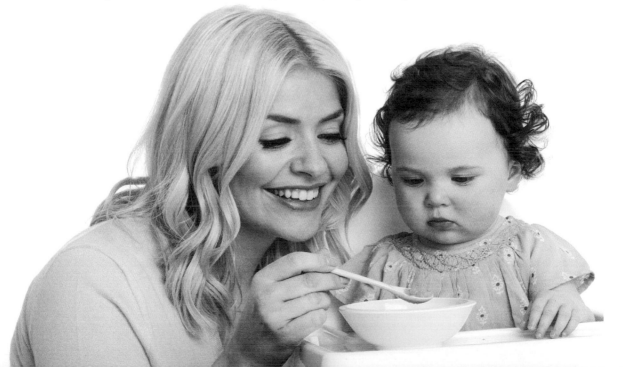

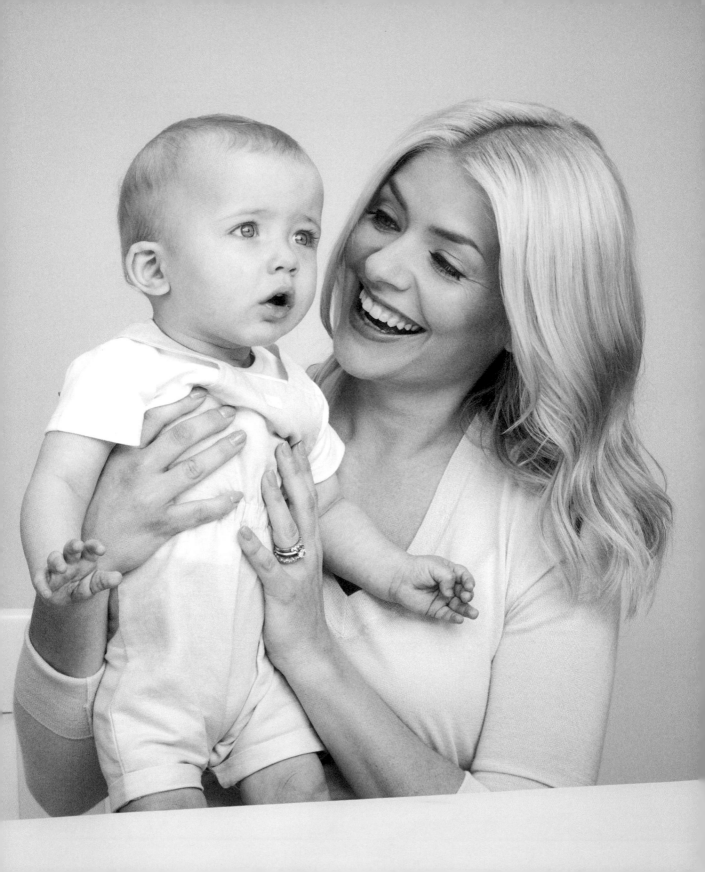

HAPPY MEALTIMES AS A FUNDAMENTAL PART OF HAPPY FAMILIES

The first few weeks of weaning aren't really conducive to the conventional family meal, given the mess and your baby's short attention span. Nevertheless, if you can, it's still important to seat your baby at the table and let her experience the whole family coming together. The early days of weaning are more exploratory for babies in terms of food, but even if you just give them an empty bowl and a spoon to practise with while you eat, they can start to copy how you use the tableware and they'll begin to feel part of the mealtime experience.

I guess every parent's dream is to have the whole family seated around the dining table, all happily tucking into the same meal you've lovingly (albeit somewhat frantically!) prepared. Basically, not having to create half a dozen different dishes to please everyone! I was really lucky growing up to have both of my parents around a lot of the time. My dad was, and still is, a salesman. His working hours used to revolve around when his customers were at home, so most days it was he who would collect me and my sister from school. We'd then all have an early dinner together as a family before he had to go out to his evening appointments.

As with so many of the good things in your own childhood, I think you only properly appreciate them when you become a parent yourself. If I'm honest, it's only since becoming a mum that I realize how lucky we were to have as much time with both our parents as we did, which is what I try to replicate for my own children. Sitting down together for a family meal is part of this. So even though Dan and my working days can be lengthy at times, we both make every effort to sit down to a family meal as often as we can and have tried to do so even during the earliest stages of weaning.

DEVELOPING GOOD EATING HABITS

In an ideal world, children will develop positive associations with everything they eat, and sharing family mealtimes as much as possible from the word go certainly helps. If you can establish this attitude from an early age, they'll by more likely to enjoy a balanced, healthy diet as they grow up. Here are a few other suggestions to encourage a good approach to eating.

VARIETY

Variety is key – the spice of life, as they say. The wider the range of different flavours, colours and textures you can introduce to children when they are young, the healthier and happier they'll be in life. Encouraging your children to be open-minded from the earliest age will help get them off to the best start nutritionally. Most babies begin with basic vegetable and fruit purées, but don't be afraid to introduce herbs, garlic and spices to widen their palate. (Not hot spices! And remember that chilli should only be introduced once your baby reaches one year old). I feel so proud of Harry and Belle now in restaurants with how receptive they are to new foods, willing to a bit more adventurous and try out other dishes rather than sticking with chicken nuggets on the kids' menu. Even when we're abroad, they always try local foods and are as partial to a seafood paella as a (not too spicy!) Thai curry.

FUSSINESS

At some point during the weaning process, you'll feel like you've got a fussy little person on your hands, and it can be frustrating, especially when the toddler stage is reached and your child suddenly realizes she can exercise control over her life. There are many reasons why this might be happening, depending on the age of your child, so before you fling some butternut squash at the kitchen wall yourself, ask yourself a few key questions:

Babies

- Is my baby hungry enough?
- Has she had too much milk at around the same time as solid feeds?
- Is she too distracted by other things at mealtime, such as the TV, toys or a busy household?
- Is she coming down with an illness?
- Is she teething?
- Is she bored of me offering the same flavours?
- Is the purée too thick for first tastes?
- Should I try mixing some of her familiar milk into the solids?

Toddlers

- Is the portion size too big and overwhelming?
- Should I try including her in meal preparation and cooking?
- Shall I try making up a meal by mixing a food I know she loves with a completely new food?
- As she rejected broccoli purée last week, should I try it a few more times? Remember that it can take up to ten goes before any given food is finally deemed acceptable!
- Shall I sit down to eat with her and let her see me eat what I'm offering her, to build up trust?

Older children

- Should I let her serve herself?
- Shall I give her the opportunity to do some cooking?
- Should I get her input for the week's meal planning?
- Shall I involve her in choosing different foods at the supermarket?

Bribery!

In the same way that one plonks the kids in front of the TV for entertainment in order to get some chores done, it's all too easy to offer something sweet as a bribe for eating a healthy main course. It's really tempting, especially if it works and gets them to eat all their veggies, and indeed needs must sometimes. But if you introduce your little one to the concept that sweet things are a reward, she might start getting the wrong attitude towards food. I regularly reward myself with junk food, for example. I think, Ooh, I've worked really hard today – I deserve a nice piece of cake! And I'm sure that attitude must stem from when I was a child, so I'm quite wary about doing the same with my kids. Somehow, I've managed to convince them that any kind of fruit or raw veg are a real treat when they're chopped up. Mango, for example, chopped-up cucumber or a peeled, sliced apple are particular favourites. They really do like those things, and not just because we don't have some fruit, such as mangoes, all the time. So, when a little bowl is offered, I can say truthfully that they find it an exciting prospect!

This is not to say my children are devoid of treats! (Indeed, Chapter 7 is all about a bit of indulgence for a special occasion.) A hot summer's day or trip to the beach needs ice cream. A cinema visit isn't the same without a tub of popcorn, and Christmas and birthdays go hand in hand with a few sweets and chocolates. But everything in moderation. If children aren't completely deprived of this sort of thing, they won't crave it and then binge once they're in the driving seat. A little bit of what you fancy does you good!

DON'T FORGET TO FEED YOURSELF HEALTHILY TOO!

Throughout the messy, time-consuming and often tiring process of weaning your baby, it can be easy to forget to look after yourself. It's crucial to remember that if you're not eating nutritionally balanced meals yourself, then you won't be getting all the energy *you* need.

The recipes in this book are all nutritionally balanced and, from Chapter 3 onwards, can be made for the whole family. If you're able (as much as possible) to enjoy meals together, then you can be certain that every member of your family (including yourself!) is getting what they need. Snacking is a slightly different matter – in times of need, when my little ones were causing havoc and it was only mid-morning – I'd sometimes be tempted by whatever cake or leftover crisps were lying around. Just try to remember that your children learn by example, so if they see you snaffling doughnuts on the sly, they might be less inclined to wolf down those veggie sticks you're offering them. You'll feel much better and more energy-filled for not turning to the high-sugar or high-salt options in times of need (although understandably it will happen now and again!)

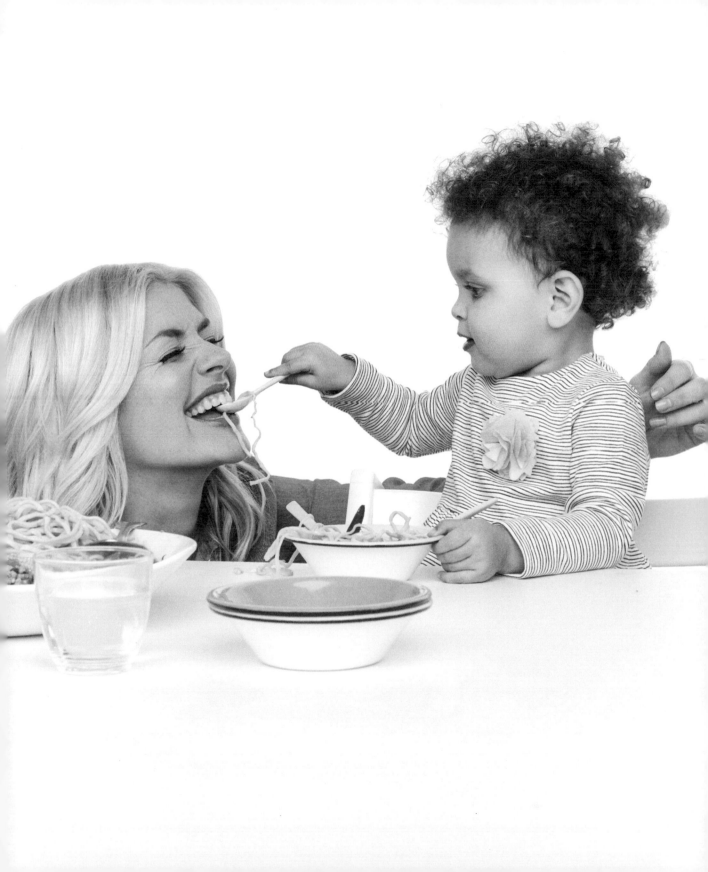

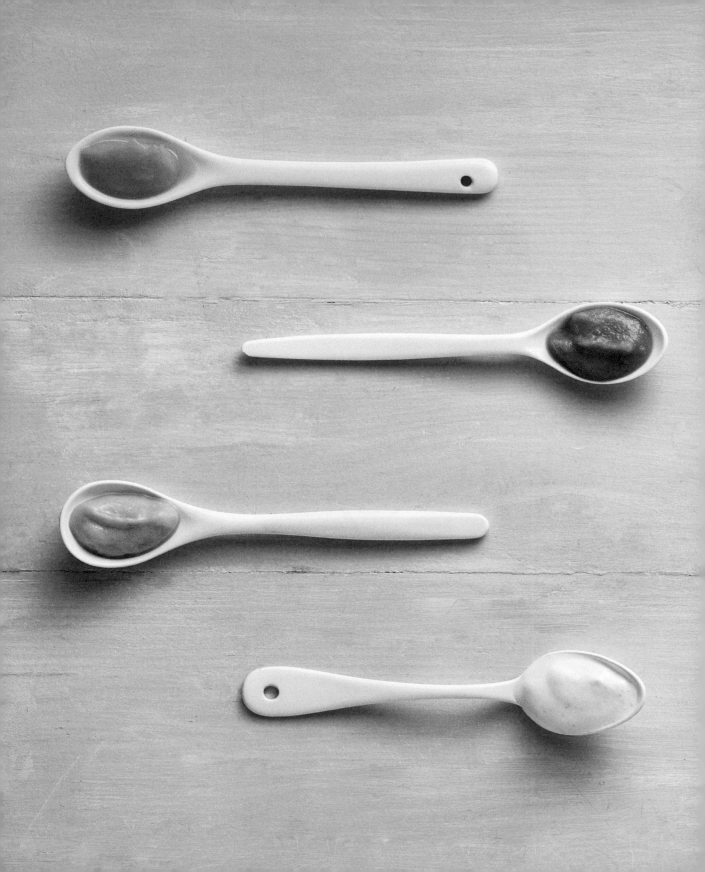

Chapter 1

6 MONTHS

WHEN TO START AND HOW TO KNOW IF YOUR BABY IS READY

Now before we embark on this journey together, the one thing I must stress is that there is no 'correct' time for you to begin the weaning process. Every baby is different, after all! And there is no rush to start your baby on solids. Equally, you should be mindful of not leaving it too late, as learning to eat solids is an important factor in your baby's motor and speech development. Plus, you might end up with a very fussy baby on your hands if you delay weaning for too long!

The most-up-to-date NHS advice recommends exclusive breast- or formula feeding up to six months, with no solids being introduced at all before that time. There are two important factors to bear in mind here. Firstly, breast milk and formula contain all the nutrients your baby needs for healthy development during the first six months of life (see page 10). And, secondly, before four months your baby's intestines and kidneys simply aren't mature enough to filter out potentially harmful substances and absorb the good bits. It's generally best to wait until six months, otherwise weaning can be harmful, leaving him at risk from infection and developing allergies. If you have a strong family history of food allergy, it's even more important you don't begin the weaning process too early, as your child may be more at risk than most.

Having said that, babies do develop at different rates and so if you believe your baby is showing all the signs of being ready (see advice on pages 40–1) then do visit your GP and get their advice. In rare cases, weaning from as early as four months can be beneficial. My GP recommended I start introducing solids to Chester from about four months, because of his severe reflux. I started him on a little baby rice for breakfast and I think the fact that it was more solid, and therefore heavier than milk, definitely helped him to keep it down. He had been in so much pain after a feed as the milk came back up, bringing the acid burn with it, I think he almost started to dread feeding, even though he was so

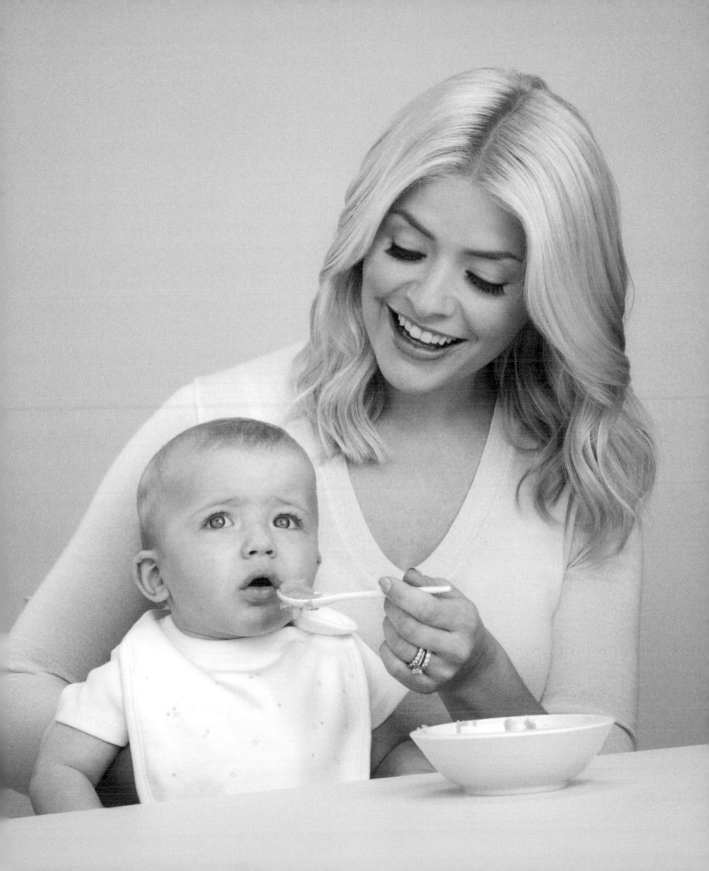

desperately hungry. I found that splitting (and eventually replacing) some milk feeds with a portion of baby rice definitely helped him through those painful few weeks. On the flip side, pre-term babies can be advised to wait between five and eight months after their birth date before starting weaning, as their internal development may be slower and therefore more immature at 4–6 months than for a baby born at full term.

In my experience – and excuse the pun – listen to your gut! You'll know if your baby is ready. All babies are different and develop at varying rates, so you are the best person to assess whether your child is ready to move on to solids. And if you feel even the slightest bit uneasy about your decision, particularly if your baby is younger than six months, then ask your GP or the health visitor for their thoughts on your individual situation. Together you'll get it right.

SIGNS THAT YOUR BABY MIGHT BE READY

Once your baby is six months old, there will be signs that he is ready to start weaning. I remember Harry and Belle just staring at me intently when we were all sitting down together at the table, watching my fork move from plate to mouth. They were completely transfixed by the action of eating – all but drooling. There are a few key signs that your baby might be ready to take to solids. They should be able to do all of these things to some capacity before you embark on weaning. Remember, though, that NHS guidelines state that milk alone is enough to sustain a baby up to six months old, so these might just indicate that he's in need of a bit more sustenance to get him through a growth spurt!

Tongue-thrust reflex

All babies are born with the tongue-thrust reflex, which prevents them from choking when they are really young. If you put something they aren't used to on their tongue, you'll see them push their tongue straight out to expel the foreign object rather than pulling it back to swallow. From about four months, this reflex starts to diminish and he'll start taking food into his mouth rather than just automatically pushing it out – this is a good sign. However, it's worth bearing in mind that even when he does start taking food into his mouth, swallowing is the next step, which might come slightly later and which is why some babies might gag initially. They don't have teeth, so they're not chewing but sucking or grinding the food between their gums until it is small enough to swallow. This is why smooth purées are among the best first foods.

Sitting up

To sit up in a feeding chair, your baby needs strong neck and head control. If you think about it, up until now you've cuddled your baby during his breast- or bottle feeds, so introducing solids while he's sitting up in a chair is a far less intimate experience for him. It's crucial that he's strong enough to hold himself upright and that he's sitting comfortably before you begin.

Reaching for food

Babies love to imitate. If you find your little one is starting to reach for things you're putting in your mouth, the chances are he's ready to have a go himself. Offering soft sticks of food is a great way of allowing him to start exploring food for himself at his own pace. See if his motor skills are developed enough for him to grab and aim the food into his mouth. (Letting your baby take the lead is the approach taken throughout baby-led weaning – see pages 182–95.) If you're spoon-feeding, you might find your baby takes more if you give him his own spoon to hold so he feels as if he's feeding himself.

HOW TO START

The secret to the whole weaning process is (where possible) to make sure the conditions are right, and this includes the feeding environment. First and foremost, brace yourself for mess! When they start weaning, babies are constantly throwing stuff on the floor and at you. You can always guarantee that the moment you do manage to get a fully loaded spoon into their mouths, they decide to sneeze it all over the table. It's a messy business, but it doesn't last for ever and, with a pack of wet wipes at the ready, rather than dealing with Armageddon in one hit at the end, you can sort it out in controlled stages.

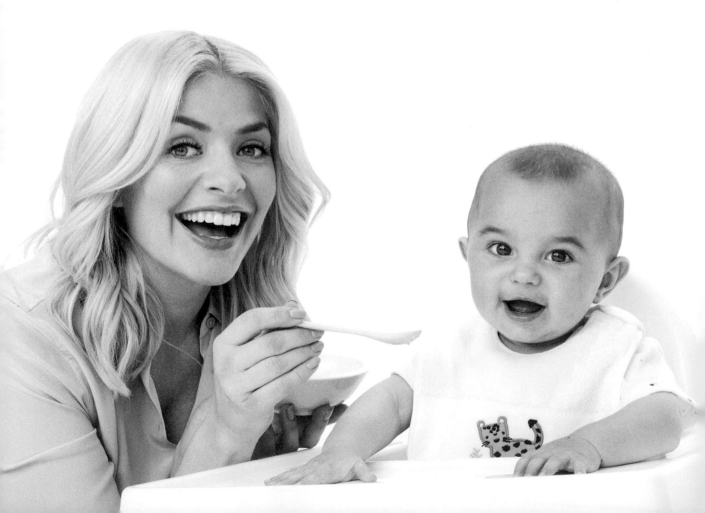

FEEDING ENVIRONMENT

Feeding chair and adjustable harness

Whether you choose a Bumbo or high chair with its own table, or one that pulls up or fixes to the dining table (see pages 27–8), the most important thing is for it to have an adjustable harness. It's imperative your baby is comfortable and well supported. If he's slouching, or there's any pressure on his tummy, it can affect feeding and lead to discomfort.

Indestructible bowl!

Any bowl that's not going to smash if it gets swiped to the floor – which, believe me, it will at some juncture! If you can bear to, allow messy play to let your baby explore for himself. Let him handle food, feel the texture and try to put it in his mouth. (For more on weaning bowls and spoons, see page 28.)

TIME OF DAY

Try to make sure your baby hasn't had too many milk feeds throughout the day, so he's hungry enough to eat. On the other hand, it's important that he's not starving when you sit him down for a meal, as he won't get the same quick fix his desperate tummy needs from a teaspoon of carrot purée as he would a bottle of milk, and the whole situation may deteriorate into a hot mess.

You need to pick a time of the day when you aren't in a rush, and most importantly when your baby is contented. With all of mine, their first ever taste of solid food was a breakfast of baby rice. I'd begin the process first thing in the morning after waking. I'd make up the usual morning bottle and a small amount of baby rice, using some of the milk from the feed. It's important to use that milk rather than additional milk, so as to avoid overfeeding. Then I'd hide the bottle from hungry little eyes, make baby comfortable in the feeding chair and offer a sip of water from a sippy cup, followed by a spoonful or so of baby rice. I'd only keep going until their interest waned and then would finish up with the usual morning bottle.

How much they eat depends entirely on your baby, but you should start to see them taking more as the days go by. Remember, it's a new and strange sensation for them, so keep the process as relaxed as possible. It's important to be guided by your baby as to how much solid food he wants and how much milk. Babies know when their tummies are full and learning to stop when they've had enough is a useful life lesson.

When you are finally sitting face to face with your baby, who's had just enough milk to appease his rumbly tummy, be prepared to melt as that first teaspoon of solid food touches his lips. There'll be a lot of gurning, tongue pushing and grimacing for the first few goes until he realizes that it's quite nice really.

At this stage, don't even expect to get more than a teaspoon's worth of food into your baby. And even that will be delivered via half a dozen spoonfuls with the tiniest amount on the edge of the spoon. Just be patient. It's all about building up your baby's confidence, taste buds and capacity for food, and it will take time for him to learn. Remember, at the earliest stages, weaning is predominantly about getting your little one familiar with food.

Texture

Initially, purées should be smooth and not too thick – about the same consistency as double cream. Start with one or two single-ingredient vegetable purées (see pages 54–5), and once your baby accepts those, then slowly introduce others. You can dilute with the vegetable-cooking water to maximize the nutrients, or with your baby's regular milk to produce something with familiar back notes.

Once you get going, you'll get a sense for what's the ideal consistency for your baby. Stick to super-smooth for the first couple of weeks, then gradually start to thicken to a consistency that doesn't quite pour off the spoon, but rather sticks to it. Think more of a mush/mash than a purée. And I mean gradually. If you try to change too soon, before he's ready, you risk a meal being rejected altogether. If your baby looks like he's starting to move the purée around his mouth, as if he's trying to chew, then it could be a sign he's ready for thicker textures. Harry loved really smooth purées; it took him longer to eat foods with lumps in it. The bottom line is not to rush it but do remember that moving on to thicker textures is important because it's good for their digestive system. Also the longer you linger on a texture the more reluctant your baby might be to move on.

Some babies will be eager to hold food and feed themselves from six months of age, while others will need a bit more encouragement. If you're allowing your little one to experiment with sticks of soft veg or fruit, the texture should be adjusted as your little one develops and they're ready for something slightly firmer and sturdier.

Breastfeeding/milk

Up until approximately six months, your baby's exclusive source of nourishment is milk (whether breast, formula or a mix) and so long as he's drinking well, keeping most of it down, and his weight is going up nicely on the scales, you can be confident he's getting all the nutrients he needs. Breast milk by its very nature is bespoke to the nutritional requirements of your baby, and the milk formulas on the market today are so highly developed, they're as close to Mum-made as possible.

It can be trickier to move an exclusively breastfed child on to solids, simply because you are removing that mother–baby intimacy, which can be a bigger wrench than for bottle-fed babies. It's a good idea to start by cutting out one of the least 'cosy' feeds and replacing it with a solid feed. Distraction is the name of the game! Don't attempt to spoon-feed your breastfed baby on your lap, as he'll immediately associate it with breastfeeding. You need to try to gradually diminish breast association as you continue to cut the milk feeds.

To begin with, your milk feeds won't change. A six-month breastfed baby will continue feeding on demand. A six-month bottle-fed baby should be having 4–5 formula feeds with a total of 840–960ml/29fl oz –1½ pints during the course of 24 hours. Once you start weaning your baby, the most important milk feeds of the day are the waking feed and last feed before bed, so make sure your baby takes full bottles at these times.

WEANING MYTHS

There are a fair few myths associated with moving your baby on to solids sooner rather than later, and I'd like to dispel them!

'The quicker you start him on solids, the quicker he'll sleep through the night.'

Babies – just like adults – wake for all sorts of reasons, and it doesn't necessarily mean they are hungry. Their tummies are so tiny in the first few months, you can't possibly hope to stuff them full enough to keep them going for hours on end. It's also worth noting that weaning coincides with a huge number of new things your baby is experiencing in his first year of life: growth spurts, teething, sitting up, crawling, walking, etc. You can put sudden changes in sleep/waking patterns down to any or all of the above. Sadly, weaning isn't a miracle cure for any of these.

'She's a big girl for five months. She needs more than milk to fill her up.'
'That baby needs to put some weight on! Give him some solids.'
'That's baby's so hungry, she's chewing her hands off! She should have some solids!'

During the early weaning stages, milk is and should still be the main source of nutrition for your baby. Whether breast or formula, milk has more calories in it than the limited amount of solid food a baby's tiny stomach can hold. Between four and eight months, weaning is more about the introduction and exploration of food and getting your little one used to the physical act of eating, rather than satisfying hunger and aiding development. If your baby appears starving at four months, try an extra milk feed before introducing solids if you feel it's too early. It might just be the top-up he needs for the moment.

VERY FIRST FOODS

At six months, keep offering the usual milk feeds. Food is merely a complement at this stage, rather than any sort of sustenance, so your baby still needs the calories and nutrition in milk.

Once you start weaning, you'll need to start giving your baby a little water at mealtimes. It's a good idea to get him used to a sippy or free flowing cup at this stage. This is a beaker with a lid and a hard spout (see page 28). It's the first step to getting your baby used to drinking from a normal lidless cup, so what better time to start than at a meal.

The following are some ideas for first foods you can try:

Baby rice

These fine, powdery flakes of rice, which you mix up in a bowl (never add to your baby's bottle) with breast milk or formula, are the perfect first taste of food. As a first solid, it's not too big a leap from what your baby will be used to flavour-wise as you're mixing it with his milk. It's also gluten-free, so allergy safe, and is fortified with vitamin B1, which helps little bodies turn the carbohydrate into energy. In the first few days, he might not take any rice down, but day by day you'll notice him take a little more, building up to a few teaspoons and maybe rejecting a milk feed completely.

Baby cereal

Baby cereals are fortified with vitamins and minerals, and most are low in sugar and salt, although be careful to check the label. In fact, be careful when selecting cereals for your children in general. It would be healthier to give them a doughnut for breakfast for all the sugar that's in some!

Vegetable purées

All the vegetables included in the recipes in Chapter 1 (see pages 54–77) are jam-packed with health-boosting nutrients. They are all excellent first foods, and most are naturally sweet and appeal to young palates. You can experiment by mixing two vegetables together, then thicken with a little baby rice or thin with your baby's usual milk, which will give it a familiar flavour. And if you're struggling with certain vegetable flavours, you can try adding a dash of apple purée or another sweet combination. This might just take the edge off any bitterness. But remember that, generally, it's best to get your baby used to vegetables before introducing sweeter, often more appealing, fruit.

Fruit purées

Babies love fruit purées (see pages 58–61). Fact. They have a naturally sweet tooth and will be drawn to all the deliciously sweet flavours. Just be careful not to overdo the fruit! It can result in a few upsets – upset tummies and the rejection of blander, savoury vegetable flavours, which is the last thing you need! Always start with a veggie purée over a fruit one.

No-cook purées

There are some fruit and veg that you don't have to cook before serving – they make wonderful first foods and are super-easy to mush up for families on the go! I'm talking about things like ripe banana, avocado, cucumber and melon. (See pages 75 and 77 for a few easy no-cook recipes.) It's a good idea to offer these even if you're not on the go to get your baby used to different textures and temperatures. You might not always have the facilities to make your baby a hot meal, so get him used to eating cold foods to avoid fussiness further down the line.

SINGLE FIRST FOODS

I've put together a few sample feeding routines for you, starting from six months. If you are weaning before then, consult your GP or midwife about what's appropriate for your little one. How you proceed safely will depend on your baby's age, weight, whether they were premature or late, etc. It's best to get medical advice, if only to confirm your gut feeling that your baby is ready.

WEEK 1

When weaning day arrived for each of mine, I tried a little baby rice at breakfast to get them started. I'd wait for them to wake up – usually around 7am – leave them with Dan for Daddy cuddles, then go to the kitchen and make up their usual morning milk feed. I'd stopped breastfeeding by six months with all of my babies, so when it was time to start weaning, they were all on formula.

Mid-morning, I'd mix up a little baby rice in a bowl, using some of the milk from the bottle, so as not to go over the quota for that feed, and prepare a sippy cup of water. For the first week, just a couple of teaspoons of baby rice is enough. When I had everything ready to go – AND HIDDEN THE BOTTLE OF MILK from hungry little eyes – I'd put them in their high chair, give them a sip of water to quench their new-day thirst and offer a little baby rice on a spoon. Not all of my children were immediately receptive to the baby rice, and I made sure I caught on camera every delicious face they pulled, but every day their interest grew, to the point that by the end of the first week, they would all manage a full teaspoon or so, before being offered the rest of their mid-morning milk feed via the bottle.

After mine got the hang of their morning baby rice, I tried a single-ingredient purée (preferably vegetable – see page 47). Mine seemed to take particularly well to Pea, Broccoli and Sweet Potato flavours (see pages 54, 56 and 57). For the first week or so, it's a good idea to mix the purée with a little of their milk feed so that it tastes vaguely familiar. I always found my children were more receptive to trying new flavours after their main nap, that is, at lunchtime. At 3pm, they're not tired and they are full of beans, bursting to see what new adventures you've got lined up for them that afternoon. As with breakfast, keep a sippy cup of water at hand to quench their thirst. You don't want to show them their milk feed until after they've had a little taste of solid food. Then, when their interest grinds to a halt, you can give them the rest of their milk feed.

SAMPLE MENU

🕐 Breakfast	Sip of water followed by baby rice and morning milk feed (175–225ml/6–8fl oz)
🕐 Mid-morning	Baby's usual milk feed (175–225ml/6–8fl oz)
🕐 Mid-afternoon	Sip of water followed by a single-ingredient purée (see pages 54–61) mixed with a little of the mid-afternoon milk feed or cooking liquor, followed by the remainder of the milk feed (175–225ml/6–8fl oz). Pea or Carrot (see page 54) are good ones to try first
🕐 Bedtime	Baby's usual milk feed (175–225ml/6–8fl oz)

What happens in Week 2 all depends on how well your baby got on in Week 1. If you didn't get much past the morning baby rice, then now's the time to start introducing his first vegetable purée. If your baby wolfed down two meals a day for most of Week 1, then you can think about adding another meal. You can also try adding an extra layer of flavour at a meal by following a purée up with some plain full-fat live yoghurt or a sweeter single-fruit purée, such as Pear, Apple, Peach or Banana (see pages 60–1). By the end of Week 2, if you are sitting him down twice a day, morning and afternoon, for solids and working in another meal around the mid-morning feed, you're well on your way to achieving three meals a day.

Be totally guided by your baby and what he can manage. If he's grouchy and fed up when you sit him down and has no desire to eat from a spoon one day, then leave it. Try again the next day. It's all about trial and error and what works best for you both.

One thing I would say is that you should try to introduce different flavours quite quickly. You can still repeat flavours, but if you're managing three sessions a day, try to make sure one of those includes something new.

SAMPLE MENU

Breakfast
Sip of water followed by baby rice mixed with some of the morning milk feed, then top up with the usual morning milk feed (175–225ml/6–8fl oz)

Mid-morning
Sip of water first, then a single-ingredient vegetable purée (see pages 54–7), followed by some plain full-fat live yoghurt. Top up with the usual mid-morning milk feed (175–225ml/6–8fl oz)

Mid-afternoon
Baby's usual milk feed (175–225ml/6–8fl oz)

Teatime
Sip of water first, then a single-ingredient vegetable purée, followed by a single-ingredient fruit purée (see pages 60–1). Try to give a different purée from the one at lunch, if possible, to encourage a varied palate

Bedtime
Baby's usual milk feed (175–225ml/6–8fl oz)

6 MONTHS

VEGETABLE PURÉES

For these first purées for your baby, it's best to start with single foods so that you can spot an allergy immediately. If there is no reaction to one kind of vegetable, then you can try another, to expand the range of different nutrients and flavours. These can also be mixed with baby cereal and/or your baby's usual milk. In addition, full-fat cow's milk can be introduced from six months as an ingredient, but not as a drink on its own in the first year. It's preferable to provide your baby with mainly veg, rather than fruit, to avoid encouraging a sweet tooth, but don't overdo the 'windy' veg, such as sprouts and cabbage.

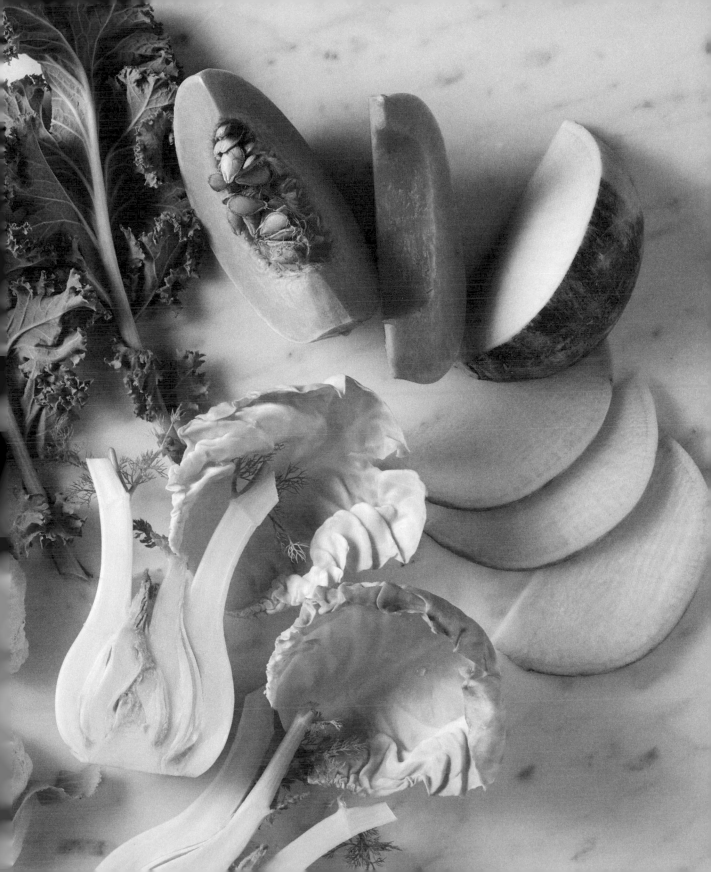

PEA

Makes 160ml/5½fl oz | ❄ *Suitable for freezing (8 ice cubes)*

125g/4½oz frozen peas

Put the peas in a saucepan and cover with water. Bring to the boil, then reduce the heat, cover the pan and simmer for 6–8 minutes or until tender. Drain over a bowl, saving 3 tablespoons of the cooking water. Place the peas and the saved water in a food processor, or use a hand blender, and purée until smooth.

PARSNIP

Makes 160ml/5½fl oz | ❄ *Suitable for freezing (8 ice cubes)*

125g/4½oz parsnip, scrubbed/peeled and cut into 1cm/½in chunks

Put the parsnip in a saucepan and cover with water. Bring to the boil, then reduce the heat, cover the pan and simmer for 10 minutes or until tender. Drain over a bowl, saving 5 tablespoons of the cooking water. Place the parsnip and the saved water in a food processor, or use a hand blender, and purée until smooth.

CARROT

Makes 120ml/4½fl oz | ❄ *Suitable for freezing (6 ice cubes)*

1 large carrot (about 100g/3½oz), scrubbed/peeled and cut into small pieces

Put the carrot in a saucepan and cover with water. Bring to the boil, then reduce the heat, cover the pan and simmer for 10 minutes or until tender. Drain over a bowl, saving 3 tablespoons of the cooking water. Place the carrot and the saved water in a food processor, or use a hand blender, and purée until smooth.

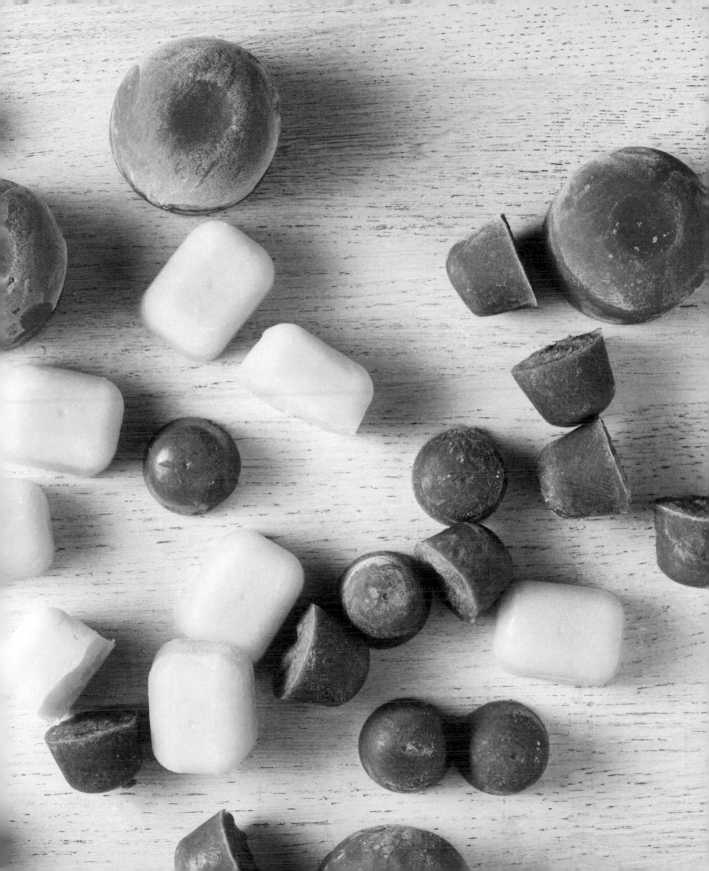

BROCCOLI

Makes 160ml/5½fl oz | ❃ *Suitable for freezing (8 ice cubes)*

100g/3½oz broccoli florets, cut into small pieces (stalks and all)

Put the broccoli in a saucepan and cover with water. Bring to the boil, then reduce the heat, cover the pan and simmer for 5–7 minutes or until tender. Drain over a bowl, saving 3 tablespoons of the cooking water. Place the broccoli and the saved water in a food processor, or use a hand blender, and purée until smooth.

COURGETTE

Makes 160ml/5½fl oz | ❃ *Suitable for freezing (8 ice cubes)*

1 courgette (about 200g/7oz), sliced (and peeled, if you like)

Put the courgette in a saucepan and cover with water. Bring to the boil, then reduce the heat, cover the pan and simmer for 3–5 minutes or until tender. Drain – as the courgette is quite watery, there is no need to save any of the cooking water – and purée until smooth in a food processor or using a hand blender.

BUTTERNUT SQUASH

Makes 200ml/7fl oz | ❃ *Suitable for freezing (10 ice cubes)*

225g/8oz butternut squash, peeled, deseeded and cut into 1cm/½in chunks

Put the squash in a saucepan and cover with water. Bring to the boil, then reduce the heat, cover the pan and simmer for 10–12 minutes or until tender. Drain over a bowl, saving 2 tablespoons of the cooking water. Place the squash and the saved water in a food processor, or use a hand blender, and purée until smooth.

SWEET POTATO

Makes 200ml/7fl oz | ❋ *Suitable for freezing (10 ice cubes)*

200g/7oz sweet potato, peeled and cut into 1cm/½in chunks

Put the sweet potato in a saucepan and cover with water. Bring to the boil, then reduce the heat, cover the pan and simmer for 10–12 minutes or until tender. Drain over a bowl, saving 3 tablespoons of the cooking water. Place the sweet potato and the saved water in a food processor, or use a hand blender, and purée until smooth.

GREEN BEAN

Makes 160ml/5½fl oz | ❋ *Suitable for freezing (8 ice cubes)*

100g/3½oz fine green beans, trimmed and quartered

Put the beans in a saucepan and cover with water. Bring to the boil, then reduce the heat, cover the pan and simmer for 8–10 minutes or until tender. Drain over a bowl, saving 2 tablespoons of the cooking water. Place the beans and the saved water in a food processor, or use a hand blender, and purée until smooth. (You may need to press the purée through a sieve for a smooth consistency.)

POTATO

Makes 200ml/7fl oz | ❋ *Suitable for freezing (10 ice cubes)*

200g/7oz potato (such as Maris Piper), peeled and cut into 1cm/½in chunks

1. Put the potato in a saucepan and cover with water. Bring to the boil, then reduce the heat, cover the pan and simmer for 12–15 minutes or until tender. Drain over a bowl, saving 3–4 tablespoons of the cooking water.
2. Transfer the potato to a bowl, then gradually add the saved water and mash between each addition until smooth. It's best to mash the potato with a fork, rather than puréeing it, as it has a tendency to become really sticky and glue-like when blended.

FRUIT PURÉES

As with the vegetable purées, start with single fruits to check for an allergic reaction. If there is no adverse reaction to one fruit, then you can try your baby on any of the purées here, and also mix them with baby cereal and/or your baby's usual milk. At this stage, be mindful of introducing citrus fruit and berries slowly as they can cause an allergic reaction.

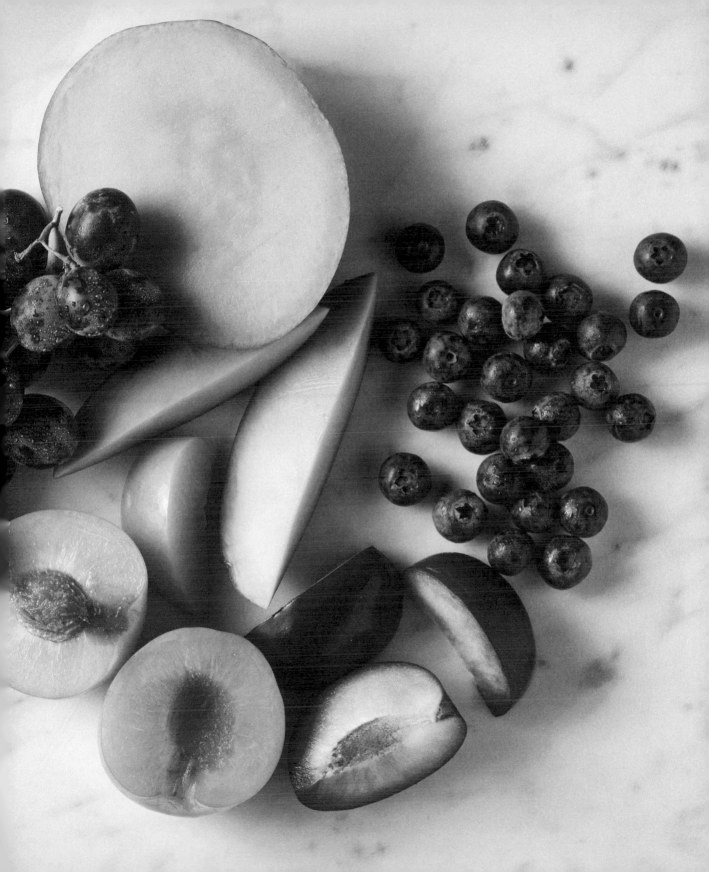

PEAR

Makes 80ml/3fl oz | ❄ *Suitable for freezing (4 ice cubes)*

1 small ripe pear (about 100g/3½oz), peeled, cored and cut into small pieces

1. If the pear is very ripe and juicy, simply purée it until smooth in a food processor or using a hand blender. You could add a splash of cooled boiled water to loosen it, if needed.
2. Alternatively, put the pear in a saucepan and cover with water. Bring to the boil, then reduce the heat, cover the pan and simmer for 5–8 minutes or until tender. Drain over a bowl, saving 1 tablespoon of the cooking water. Purée the pear until smooth, adding the saved water if needed, in a food processor or using a hand blender.

PEACH

Makes 80ml/3fl oz | ❄ *Suitable for freezing (4 ice cubes)*

1 ripe peach

1. To remove the skin, put the peach in a heatproof bowl. Pour over enough just-boiled water to cover and leave for 1 minute for very ripe fruit (or up to 5 minutes if the peach is slightly firm). Using a slotted spoon, remove the peach and rinse under cold running water until cool enough to handle. Peel off the skin, cut in half and remove the stone.
2. Purée the peach until smooth, adding a splash of cooled boiled water if needed, in a food processor or using a hand blender.

APPLE

Makes 120ml/4½fl oz | ❊ *Suitable for freezing (6 ice cubes)*

1 eating apple (about 100g/3½oz), peeled, cored and cut into small pieces

Put the apple in a saucepan and cover with water. Bring to the boil, then reduce the heat, cover the pan and simmer for 8–10 minutes or until tender. Drain over a bowl, saving 3 tablespoons of the cooking water. Place the apple and the saved water in a food processor, or use a hand blender, and purée until smooth.

PAPAYA

Makes 80ml/3fl oz | ❊ *Suitable for freezing (4 ice cubes)*

1 ripe papaya, peeled, halved and the seeds scooped out

Purée the papaya until smooth in a food processor or using a hand blender, adding a splash of cooled boiled water, if needed.

BANANA

Makes 60ml/2½fl oz | ❊ *Suitable for freezing (3 ice cubes)*

1 small ripe banana, peeled

Using the back of a fork or a hand blender, mash the banana until smooth, adding a splash of cooled boiled water, if needed.

AVOCADO

Makes 80ml/3fl oz

Flesh of 1 small ripe avocado

Using the back of a fork or a hand blender, mash the avocado until smooth, adding a splash of cooled boiled water, if needed. This purée is best made just before serving as the avocado is prone to lose its colour if prepared too far in advance.

COMBINING FIRST FOODS

By Week 3 and certainly into Week 4, you will hopefully be going great guns. If you think your baby is coping well with the smooth purées, you can start to think about thicker, combined ones. For thicker purées, you can use less of the cooking water or your baby's milk, or a little more baby rice.

In an ideal world, the quicker he learns to manage thicker textures, the less fussy he'll be further down the road. On pages 64–77, you'll find some of my favourite combined purées, such as Parsnip and Pear (see page 68) and Garden Veg (see page 64). Mixing ingredients together like this will help your baby get used to flavour combinations. And don't forget to try some no-cook purées, such as Avocado and Pear (see page 75), as this will add more texture variants to your baby's diet.

One of the main pieces of advice I can give you at this stage is to move your baby through the stages quite quickly – ideally, he'll be moving quite large but soft lumps around his mouth by about seven or eight months. My sister, who didn't do this, found it much harder to get her daughter to progress from smooth purées as she panicked every time Lola appeared to gag on a lump. They all do it; it's part of the learning process. Just as they learn to 'gum' the lump a bit smaller next time, to help it go down. Moving them through the texture changes is a case of gentle perseverance. Don't force the issue, but keep trying! They'll get there.

SAMPLE MENU

🕐 **Breakfast**   Sip of water followed by baby rice mixed with some of the morning milk feed, then top up with the usual morning milk feed (175–225ml/6–8fl oz)

🕐 **Mid-morning**   Sip of water followed by a combination purée, such as Broccoli, Courgette and Rice (see page 69). A no-cook purée is great if you're out and about, such as Cucumber, Melon and Mint (see page 75). Top up with the usual mid-morning milk feed (175–225ml/6–8fl oz)

🕐 **Mid-afternoon**   Baby's usual milk feed (175–225ml/ 6–8fl oz)

🕐 **Teatime**   Sip of water followed by a combination purée, such as Sweet Potato and Cauliflower (see page 69). You could try some Pear or Apple purée (see pages 60 and 61) combined with plain full-fat live yoghurt as a dessert

🕐 **Bedtime**   Baby's usual milk feed (175–225ml/6–8fl oz)

GREEN BEAN AND APPLE

Makes 320ml/11fl oz | ❋ *Suitable for freezing (16 ice cubes)*

Babies naturally have a sweet tooth, but it's a good idea to get them familiar with vegetables and savoury flavours from the get-go. This simple purée may ease them in.

50g/2oz fine green beans, trimmed and thinly sliced

2 eating apples, peeled, cored and cut into small pieces

2 tbsp plain full-fat live yoghurt

1. Put the green beans and apples in a small saucepan and cover with water. Bring to the boil, then turn the heat down slightly and simmer, covered, for 6–8 minutes until tender. Drain over a bowl, saving 2 tablespoons of the cooking water.
2. Purée the beans and apples with the saved water and yoghurt in a food processor, or using a hand blender, until smooth.

GARDEN VEG

Makes 280ml/10fl oz | ❋ *Suitable for freezing (14 ice cubes)*

The potato and milk add a comforting creaminess to this purée, helping to tame the stronger flavour of the leek.

150g/5oz potato (such as Maris Piper), peeled and cut into 1cm/½in chunks

60g/2½oz frozen peas

1 small leek (about 60g/2½oz), finely chopped

3 tbsp baby's usual milk

1. Put the potato in a saucepan and cover with water. Bring to the boil, then reduce the heat, cover the pan and simmer for 10 minutes. Add the peas and leek, and cook for 5 more minutes or until tender.
2. Place the vegetables and milk in a food processor, or use a hand blender, and purée until smooth.

CREAMY PEAR AND RICE

Makes 100ml/3½fl oz

If you're planning to move on from single-ingredient purées, then this is a great one to start with. The cinnamon adds a touch of natural sweetness, though you can leave it out, if you prefer. As a precautionary measure during weaning, I don't recommend keeping leftover cooked rice as it's important to be incredibly careful when reheating it, due to the slight risk of food poisoning.

15g/½oz white long-grain rice, rinsed

½ ripe pear, peeled, cored and cut into pieces

1–2 tbsp baby's usual milk

Pinch of ground cinnamon (optional)

1. Put the rice in a small saucepan, cover with water and bring to the boil. Turn the heat down to low, cover the pan and simmer for 12–15 minutes or until the rice is cooked, adding the pear 5 minutes before the end of the cooking time. (If the pear is very ripe, you can simply purée it with the cooked rice.)
2. Place the rice, the smaller quantity of milk and the cinnamon (if using) in a food processor, or use a hand blender, and purée until smooth. Add the remaining milk if the purée is too thick.

BABY BLUEBERRY PORRIDGE

Makes 240ml/8½fl oz | ❋ *Suitable for freezing (12 ice cubes)*

This recipe is so simple and was a favourite for each of my little ones. I used frozen blueberries as they have a softer texture and skin, so are easier to blend; a bag kept in the freezer is also very convenient. You can use fresh berries otherwise.

25g/1oz rolled porridge oats

250ml/9fl oz baby's usual milk, plus extra if needed

50g/2oz frozen (or fresh) blueberries

Large pinch of ground flaxseeds/linseeds (optional)

1. Put the oats in a bowl with the milk and leave them to soak overnight, or for a minimum of 1 hour if you don't have more time. (While not essential, soaking the oats not only speeds up the cooking time but is also believed to make them easier to digest.)

2. The next day, tip the soaked oat mixture into a saucepan and stir in the blueberries. Place over a medium-high heat and when the porridge just starts to bubble, turn the heat down to low and cook, stirring, for 10 minutes or until the oats are very tender.

3. Purée the porridge until smooth in a food processor or using a hand blender. This may take a little time – do add a splash more milk if it's too thick. Stir in the ground flaxseeds, if using, at the end.

» Most large supermarkets and health-food shops now sell ground flaxseeds – also known as linseeds. A sprinkling is a great way of boosting intake of heart-friendly omega-3 fatty acids. However, if there is any history of nut or seed allergy in the family, they are best avoided for now.

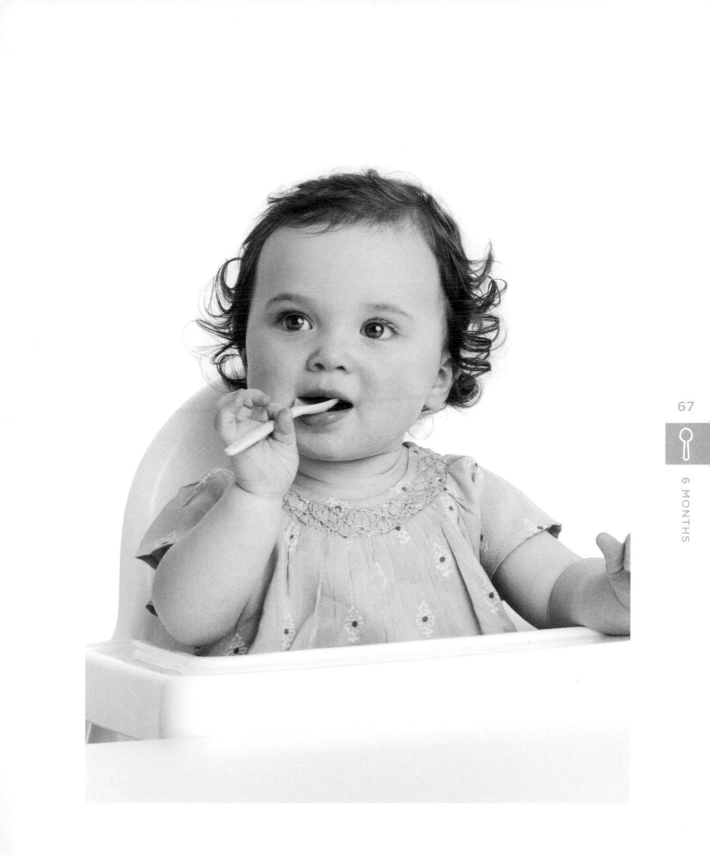

DRIED APRICOT AND RICE

Makes 125ml/4½fl oz

Try to use dark-coloured dried apricots rather than the bright orange ones, which contain the preservative sulphur, possibly thought to aggravate asthma symptoms in susceptible individuals. Dark apricots have a delicious sticky texture and almost toffee-like flavour. Check the packet label to make sure they are unsulphured.

15g/½oz unsulphured dark dried apricots, chopped

15g/½oz white long-grain rice, rinsed

3–4 tbsp baby's usual milk

1. Put the apricots and rice in a saucepan, cover with water and bring to the boil. Turn the heat down to low, cover the pan and simmer for 12–15 minutes or until the rice is cooked. Drain the rice and apricots.
2. Place the apricots, rice and the smaller quantity of milk in a food processor, or use a hand blender, and purée until smooth. Add the remaining milk if the purée is too thick.

PARSNIP AND PEAR

Makes 200ml/7fl oz | ❄ *Suitable for freezing (10 ice cubes)*

Parsnip can be an acquired taste, but partner it with pear and it's transformed. This purée is also surprisingly good with roast pork as an alternative to the usual apple sauce.

125g/4½oz parsnip, peeled and cut into 1cm/½in chunks

1 small ripe pear, peeled, cored and cut into 1.5cm/⅝in chunks

1. Put the parsnip and pear in a saucepan, and cover with water. Bring to the boil, then reduce the heat and simmer for 8–10 minutes or until tender. Drain over a bowl, saving 2 tablespoons of the cooking water.
2. Place the parsnip, pear and saved water in a food processor, or use a hand blender, and purée until smooth.

BROCCOLI, COURGETTE AND RICE

Makes 175ml/6fl oz

Eggs are a good source of vitamin D, which is essential for normal teeth and bone development. Just the yolk is used here as it combines more easily with the rest of the ingredients, but you could use the white as well.

15g/½oz white long-grain rice, rinsed

25g/1oz broccoli florets, cut into small pieces (stalks and all)

1 small courgette, cut into large chunks

Large pinch of dried mint (optional)

1 hard-boiled egg yolk

1. Put the rice in a saucepan and cover with water. Bring to the boil, then turn the heat down to low, cover the pan and simmer for 7–8 minutes. Add the broccoli, courgette and mint, if using, and cook for another 5 minutes or until all are tender. Drain over a bowl, saving 3–4 tablespoons of the cooking water.
2. Place the rice, vegetables, egg yolk and the smaller quantity of saved water in a food processor, or use a hand blender, and purée until smooth. Add the remaining water, if needed.

SWEET POTATO AND CAULIFLOWER

Makes 240ml/8½fl oz | ❄ *Suitable for freezing (12 ice cubes)*

Babies are particularly sensitive to bitter vegetables such as cauliflower, broccoli and green leaves, but if you combine them with dairy foods and sweeter veg, including sweet potatoes, you dilute any bitterness and make them more palatable to your child.

125g/4½oz sweet potato, peeled and cut into 1cm/½in chunks

50g/2oz cauliflower florets, cut into small pieces (stalks and all)

100ml/3½fl oz baby's usual milk

1. Put the sweet potato in a saucepan and cover with water. Bring to the boil, then reduce the heat, cover the pan and simmer for 5 minutes. Add the cauliflower and cook for another 5–7 minutes or until tender.
2. Place the vegetables and milk in a food processor, or use a hand blender, and purée until smooth.

BLUEBERRY, APPLE AND SPINACH

Makes 200ml/7fl oz | ❄ *Suitable for freezing (10 ice cubes)*

If you're struggling to get your baby to eat green veg, which is inherently bitter, then combining it with fruit may help. In this purée, the vitamin C present in the blueberries and apple helps the body absorb the iron in the spinach more efficiently. Frozen blueberries are used for easier blending, though you could use fresh ones instead.

1 eating apple, peeled, cored and cut into small pieces

100g/3½oz frozen (or fresh) blueberries

15g/½oz baby leaf spinach

1. Put the apple in a saucepan with 2 tablespoons of water and cook over a medium heat for 5 minutes. Add the blueberries and spinach, and cook for another 3 minutes or until everything is tender.
2. Place the apple, blueberries and spinach, along with any water left in the pan, in a food processor, or use a hand blender, and purée until smooth. Add a splash of cooled boiled water, if needed.

APPLE AND SWEET POTATO

Makes 200ml/7fl oz | ❄ *Suitable for freezing (10 ice cubes)*

Bright and cheering, this makes a vibrant golden purée. Sweet potato is a great source of vitamin A, which is essential for healthy eyes and skin. The small amount of butter in the dish helps the body absorb this vitamin.

125g/4½oz sweet potato, peeled and cut into 1cm/½in chunks

1 eating apple, peeled, cored and cut into small pieces

5g/¼oz unsalted butter

1. Put the sweet potato in a saucepan and cover with water. Bring to the boil, then reduce the heat and simmer for 5 minutes. Add the apple and cook for another 5–8 minutes or until both the apple and sweet potato are tender. Drain over a bowl, saving 3 tablespoons of the cooking water.
2. Place the sweet potato and apple with the butter and saved water in a food processor, or use a hand blender, and purée until smooth.

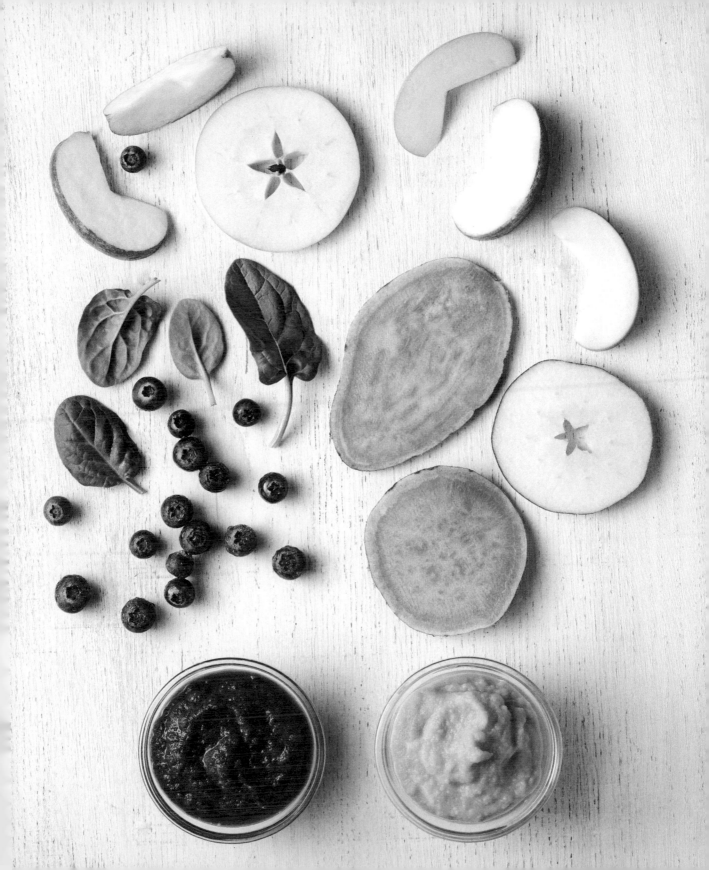

SQUASH AND RED LENTIL

Makes 240ml/8½fl oz | *❋ Suitable for freezing (12 ice cubes)*

Lentils are a good vegetarian source of iron, your baby's stores of which start to decline at around six months. That said, lentils should only be given in small amounts as they are high in soluble fibre, which can fill a baby's stomach up quickly, stopping him from getting all the nutrients he needs.

25g/1oz split red lentils, rinsed

225g/8oz butternut squash, peeled, deseeded and cut into 1cm/½in chunks

3–4 tbsp baby's usual milk (optional)

1. Put the lentils in a saucepan and cover with water. Bring to the boil and cook for 10 minutes. Add the squash and cook for another 10 minutes or until tender and the lentils are starting to break down. Drain over a bowl, saving 3–4 tablespoons of the cooking water, if not using the milk.
2. Place the lentils, squash and the smaller quantity of milk, if using, or saved water in a food processor, or use a hand blender, and purée until smooth. Add the remaining milk or water, if needed.

RED CABBAGE, PEAR AND SWEET POTATO

Makes 320ml/11fl oz | *❋ Suitable for freezing (16 ice cubes)*

This may sound like a quirky combination of ingredients, but they work well together as well as providing a range of vitamins and minerals. If the pear is ripe enough it won't need cooking, but if yours is still a little firm, cook it with the sweet potato and cabbage for 5 minutes until tender.

150g/5oz sweet potato, peeled and cut into 1cm/½in chunks

50g/2oz red cabbage, thinly sliced

1 ripe pear, peeled, cored and chopped

4–5 tbsp baby's usual milk

Put the sweet potato and cabbage in a saucepan, and cover with water. Bring to the boil, then reduce the heat, cover the pan and simmer for 10–12 minutes or until tender. Drain and place in a food processor with the pear and the smaller quantity of milk, or use a hand blender. Blend until smooth, adding the remaining milk, if needed.

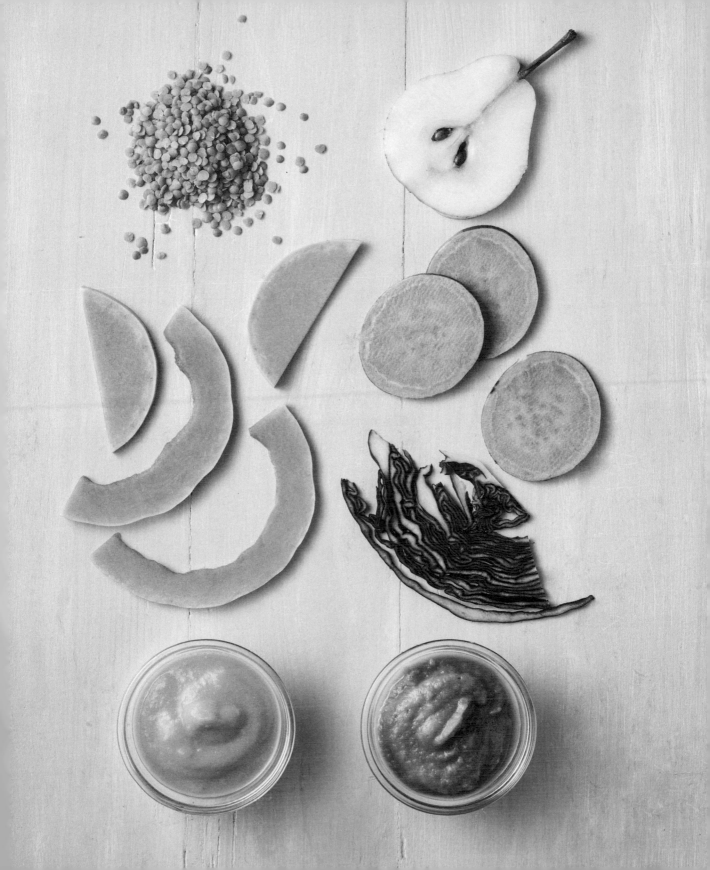

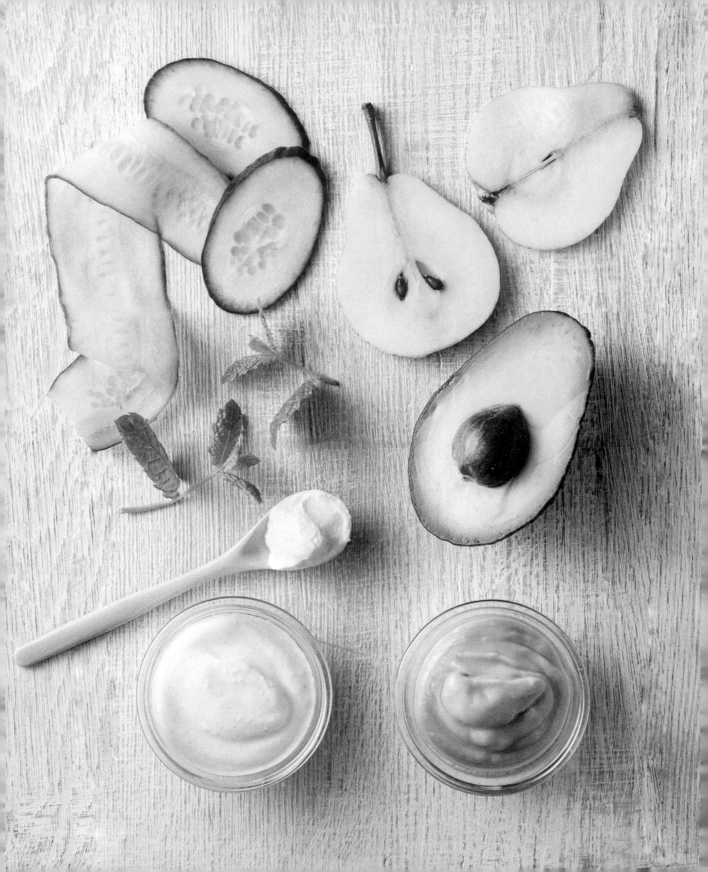

AVOCADO AND PEAR

Makes 90ml/3¼fl oz

Avocado adds a rich creaminess to this purée as well as beneficial fats and the antioxidant vitamin E. It's best made just before serving to keep its green colour, but a squeeze of fresh lemon juice helps slow down discoloration, if you want to keep the purée for longer.

1 small ripe pear, peeled, cored and cut into small pieces

Flesh of ½ small ripe avocado

Squeeze of lemon juice (optional)

Place the pear and avocado in a food processor, or use a hand blender, and purée until smooth. Add the lemon juice to stop the purée turning brown, if not serving straight away.

CUCUMBER, MELON AND MINT

Makes 120ml/4½fl oz | ❋ *Suitable for freezing (6 ice cubes)*

A taste of summer! If your melon is extra juicy, use slightly less of it or the purée will be quite runny. It also makes nifty little ice-cube pops for older babies – just pour the purée into an ice-cube tray and insert a lolly stick into each hole of the tray before freezing.

40g/1½oz honeydew melon flesh, chopped

2.5cm/1in piece of cucumber, peeled, deseeded and chopped

5 fresh mint leaves

3 tbsp plain full-fat live Greek yoghurt

Place the melon, cucumber, mint and yoghurt in a food processor, or use a hand blender, and purée until smooth.

BROCCOLI, AVOCADO AND CHEESE

Makes 125ml/4½fl oz

When it comes to weaning, avocados are a blessing. Super-nutritious, they also make a lovely creamy purée in next to no time. The only downside is that they turn brown soon after cutting, so this is best made just before serving.

25g/1oz broccoli florets, cut into small pieces (stalks and all)

Flesh of ½ small ripe avocado

8g/⅓oz mature Cheddar cheese, grated

3 tbsp baby's usual milk

Put the broccoli in a saucepan and cover with water. Bring to the boil, then reduce the heat, cover the pan and simmer for 5 minutes until tender. Drain and place in a food processor with the avocado, Cheddar and milk, or use a hand blender, and purée until smooth.

KALE, RICE AND PEAS

Makes 240ml/8½fl oz

The addition of egg yolk bumps up the protein and vitamin A content of this purée. You could also add the egg white, but I think it tastes (and looks) better with just the yolk – just make sure the egg is completely cooked, and there is no trace of runniness.

25g/1oz white long-grain rice, rinsed

15g/½oz kale leaves, finely chopped

60g/2½oz frozen peas

1 hard-boiled egg yolk

1. Put the rice in a saucepan and cover with water. Bring to the boil, then turn the heat down to low, cover the pan and simmer for 7 minutes. Add the kale and peas to the pan, stir, cover again with the lid and simmer for another 5–7 minutes or until everything is cooked. Drain over a bowl, saving 7–8 tablespoons of the cooking water.
2. Place the rice, vegetables and the smaller quantity of saved water in a food processor, or use a hand blender, and purée until smooth. Add the remaining water, if needed.

BANANA, YOGHURT AND AVOCADO

Makes 90ml/3¼fl oz

This tastes great as it is, but it also makes a surprisingly good, healthy chocolate mousse for anyone over a year old. Simply blend in a tablespoon each of cocoa or cacao powder and a little maple syrup or honey (babies shouldn't be given honey or added sugar before a year old, but if you use a really sweet, overripe banana you won't need any extra sweetener) and you're done.

1 small ripe banana, peeled

Flesh of ¼ avocado

1 tbsp plain full-fat live yoghurt

Squeeze of lemon juice (optional)

Place the banana, avocado and yoghurt in a food processor, or use a hand blender, and purée until smooth. Add the lemon juice to stop the purée turning brown, if not serving straight away.

SLEEPY-TIME LETTUCE AND BANANA

Makes 80ml/3fl oz | ❄ *Suitable for freezing (4 ice cubes)*

Both lettuce and bananas are said to have sleep-inducing properties, and this purée may be worth a try if your baby is struggling to get enough restful sleep. Serve it about 2 hours before sleep-time.

1 small ripe banana, peeled and sliced

15g/½oz butterhead lettuce leaves

1 tbsp baby's usual milk

Using a food processor or hand blender, purée the banana, lettuce and milk until smooth.

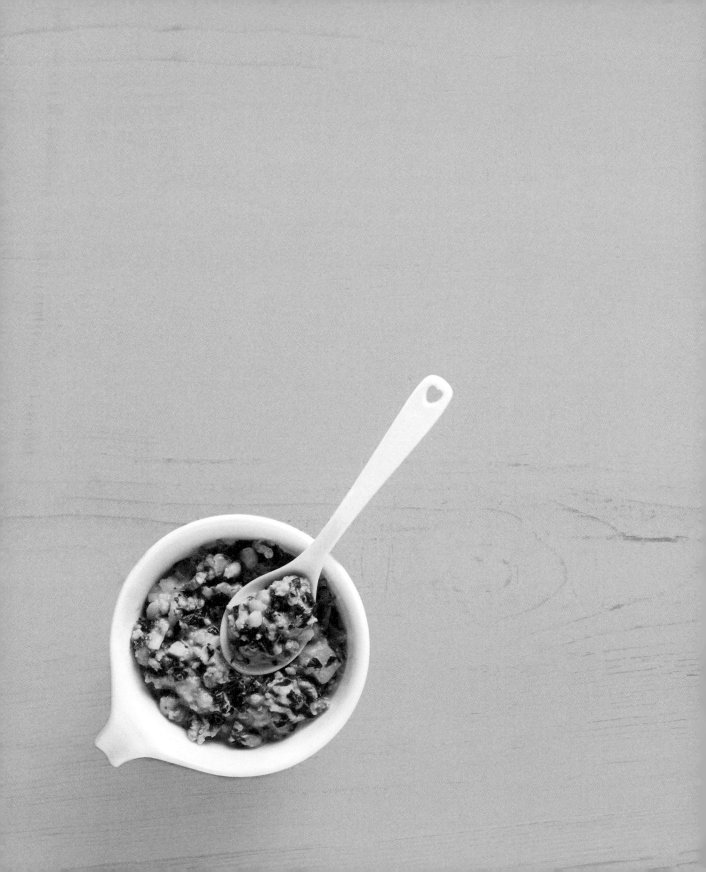

Chapter 2

7-9 MONTHS

After the first month or so of weaning, your baby will still be getting more food on herself and the floor than in her tummy. Hopefully, she'll be getting used to the idea of having more than just milk and if she is responding well and enjoying the purées, then keep going and try some of the recipes in this chapter. The name of the game is to up the texture, variety and quantity without her noticing any sudden change.

If your baby has been a little slower on the uptake, be guided by her – but don't give in completely. It's important to keep offering purées, even if she only takes the smallest amount each time. She'll soon get used to it and trust you. Babies, like adults, can be wary of new experiences and you need to have patience and earn their trust.

HOW MUCH TO FEED YOUR BABY

Quantities at this stage will be dependent on how quickly your baby is taking to weaning, and how well she adapts to the introduction of other foods. Generally, I'd advise that mealtimes should consist of between 3 and 9 teaspoons of purée per meal. Your baby's stomach capacity will have grown a bit since you first started weaning, but remember that if you're serving more protein- and carbohydrate-rich foods, she will become full more quickly.

Gluten-based foods like pasta and bread take quite a lot of digesting, so don't overload your early feeder. Offering them once a day is enough until her digestive system is more developed, or avoid gluten altogether until she's older, if you think she might be reacting badly.

Also, don't be tempted to give your baby whole grains like brown pasta, brown bread and brown rice. It might feel like you're doing the healthy thing, but babies don't need as much fibre as adults do. It can fill them up too much and prevent them from having enough room to take in other vital nutrients. It can also deplete them of minerals if their bowels are over-stimulated.

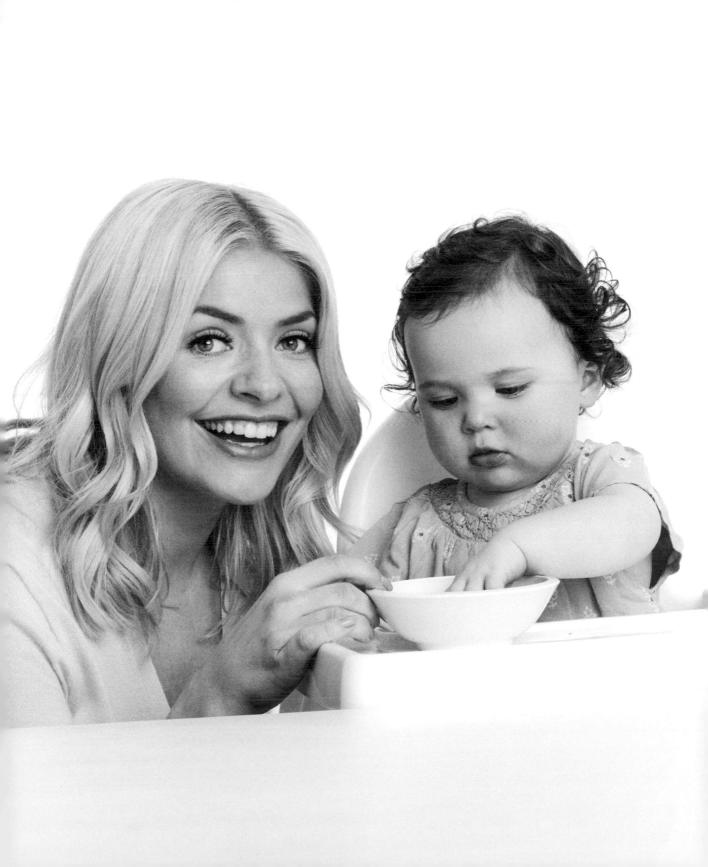

Every baby is different, so there's no set timetable to follow when you move from super-smooth purées to mush and then to chopped food. You need to be guided by your baby's response to tasting, eating and swallowing, and move through the textural stages as swiftly as your baby's response permits. If she's responding well, and you think she's nailed mush, make the lumps a bit bigger by briefly mashing or mushing food instead of whizzing it finely. You might also want to try introducing more baby rice, grating in soft vegetables or even adding small lumps, such as baby pasta shapes (e.g. Chicken Minestrone or Pasta with Courgette and Cheese on pages 103 and 92), oats (e.g. Carrot and Apricot Porridge on page 86), couscous or quinoa (e.g. Lamb and Apricot Couscous on page 102). Your baby may also be ready to start feeding herself finger foods using her hands.

Warning: At this stage, your baby will gag at some point! To reassure you, gagging is quite vocal whereas choking tends to happen silently. I will warn you now that gagging doesn't just stop overnight and will become a regular mealtime occurrence. Only once her tongue-thrust reflex (see page 41) has relaxed completely will she begin to learn how to move food from the front to the back of her mouth. Toothless chewing, or gumming, is the way babies break down the larger lumps of food and thicker textures they're receiving. However, it takes a while to master the art of swallowing, so your baby will sometimes gag when she eats. In fact, every time you up the texture of her purées, be prepared for gagging. The first time you see it, it's horrendous – you panic and think, Oh my God, what have I done! Try not to leap up from the table to immediately turn your child upside down, as gagging is a perfectly normal and natural safety mechanism that prevents your little one from choking.

INTRODUCING FOODS GRADUALLY

As you start to introduce more ingredients, you are likely to be wary of allergies. The way to check for them is not to introduce too many foods at once. Once you're sure your baby has responded well to a particular flavour or food group, move on to the next.

BREASTFEEDING/MILK

Remember: a baby still needs 500–600ml/18fl oz–1 pint of milk across her daily feeds up until she is a year old. However, it's only natural that the more solid food a baby consumes, the less milk she will want. At around 8–9 months, all of mine dropped the mid-morning milk feed.

At this stage, milk is still a baby's main source of vital nutrients. So if you find your baby is really off her milk when you start introducing more lumpy/ substantial purées and meals, be patient and keep on offering it. You should use as much of the milk quota in your cooking as possible to make sure she's still getting the nutrients she needs. If your baby gets ill, however, the first thing to go will be her appetite for solids, and you should reinstate full milk feeds until she starts to get better and wants food again.

Finally, remember to give your baby a sippy cup with a lid (see page 28) filled with tap water at mealtimes. Don't be tempted to give bottled water as this tends to contain too many minerals and salts.

SAMPLE MENU

🕐 **Breakfast** Sip of water followed by Orchard Fruit Oats (see page 89) or Tomato Quinoa Bowl (see page 90). Top up with milk feed

🕐 **Mid-morning** Baby's usual milk feed

🕐 **Lunch** Sip of water followed by Spiced Squash, Lentil and Apple (see page 95) or Easy Chicken Tagine (see page 100). Ideally something you've batch-cooked that requires no prep time whatsoever! Possibly with a few cooked soft vegetable sticks to get baby used to finger feeding.

🕐 **Afternoon** Baby's usual milk feed

🕐 **Teatime** Sip of water followed by Baby 'Baked' Beans (see page 93) or Simple Spaghetti Bolognese (see page 96). Follow up with a few pieces of fresh fruit such as pear or watermelon.

🕐 **Bedtime** Baby's usual milk feed

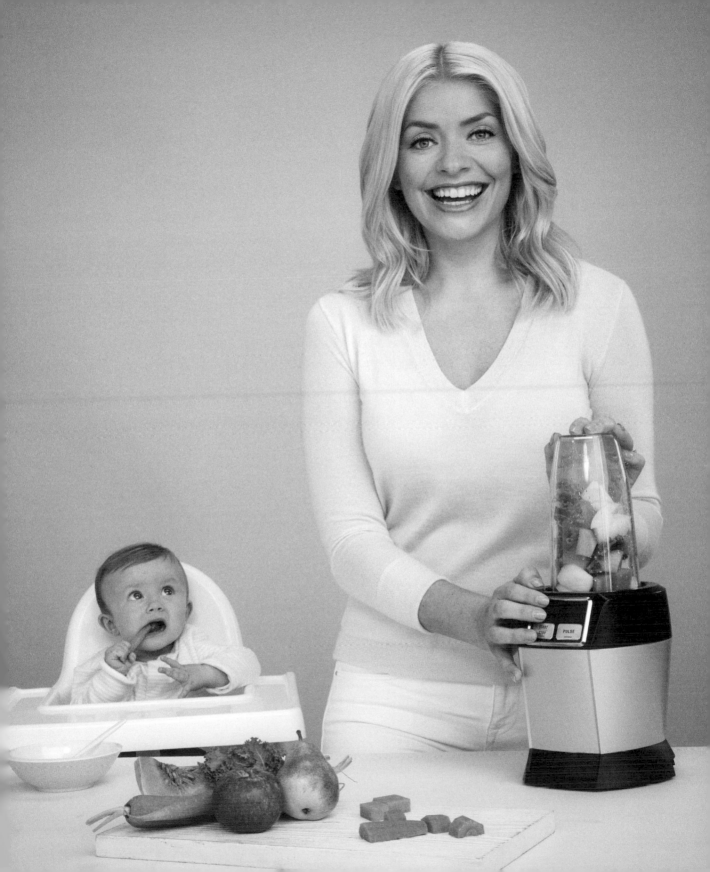

CARROT AND APRICOT PORRIDGE

Makes 280ml/10fl oz (2–4 portions) | ❄ *Suitable for freezing (14 ice cubes)*

This is a simple way to boost the quantity of veg your baby eats. While soaking the oats isn't essential, it does speed up the cooking time and is believed to make them easier to digest. Apricots are a good source of iron, but be sure to use the dark, unsulphured ones.

25g/1oz rolled porridge oats

25g/1oz unsulphured dark dried apricots, roughly chopped

350ml/12fl oz full-fat milk, plus extra if needed

2 tbsp finely grated carrot

Pinch of ground cinnamon (optional)

1. Put the oats and apricots in a bowl with the milk and leave them to soak overnight, or for a minimum of 1 hour, if you don't have more time.
2. The next day, tip the soaked oat mixture into a saucepan and stir in the carrot. Bring almost to the boil, then turn the heat down to low and simmer, stirring constantly, for 10 minutes or until cooked through, adding a splash more milk, if needed. Stir in the cinnamon, if using.
3. Using the back of a fork, mash to a coarse purée. Alternatively, blend in a food processor or using a hand blender.

APPLE AND BLUEBERRY BREAKFAST

Makes 160ml/5½fl oz (1–2 portions) | ❄ *Suitable for freezing (8 ice cubes)*

You should be able to find ground flaxseeds/linseeds in most large supermarkets and health-food shops. They are a valuable vegetarian source of heart- and brain-supporting omega-3 fatty acids, and a sprinkling is virtually undetectable in this breakfast. Look for plain full-fat live yoghurt, which contains beneficial bacteria that boost the health of the gut.

⅓ quantity of Blueberry, Apple and Spinach (see page 70)

4 tbsp thick plain full-fat live yoghurt

¼ tsp ground flaxseeds/linseeds (optional)

Mix together all the ingredients in a bowl and serve when ready.

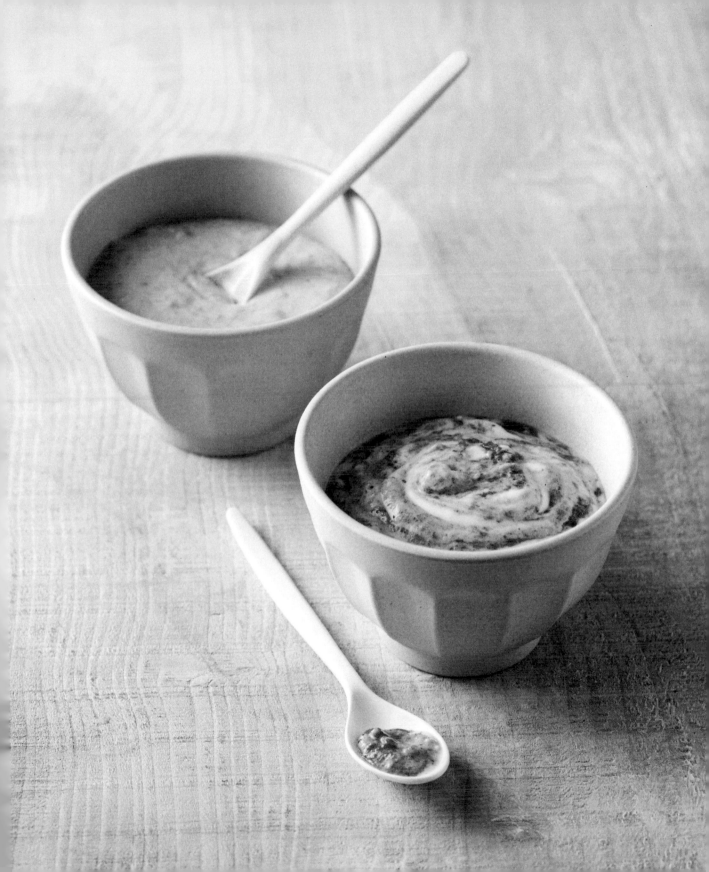

MANGO, RICE AND EGG

Makes 200ml/7fl oz (2–3 portions)

Recently, there's been a lot in the news about the immune-boosting properties of vitamin D or the 'sunshine vitamin'. It can be hard to get enough during the winter months, so it's worth upping dietary sources, such as egg yolk.

25g/1oz white long-grain rice, rinsed

100g/3½oz ripe mango flesh, chopped

1 hard-boiled egg yolk

4 tbsp full-fat milk, plus extra if needed

Pinch of ground cinnamon

1. Put the rice in a saucepan, cover with water and bring to the boil. Turn the heat down to low, cover the pan and simmer for 10–12 minutes or until tender, then drain.
2. Place the rice, mango, egg yolk, milk and cinnamon in a food processor, or use a hand blender, and purée until smooth and creamy. Add a splash more milk, if needed.

BANANA, GINGER AND PEAR

Makes 320ml/11fl oz (2–4 portions) | ❊ *Suitable for freezing (16 ice cubes)*

A tummy-soothing combination of banana, plain full-fat live yoghurt and ginger. Dried ginger, in particular, is believed to help settle the stomach – only a pinch is used here, mind you, since it does provide a blast of heat.

1 ripe pear, peeled, cored and chopped

½ small ripe banana, peeled and chopped

50g/2oz slice of good-quality white bread, crusts removed, torn into small pieces

3–4 tbsp full-fat milk

3 tbsp thick plain full-fat live yoghurt

Pinch of ground ginger

1. If the pear is a little hard, cook it first in boiling water for 5–8 minutes or until tender, then drain.
2. Put the pear in a food processor with the banana, bread, the smaller quantity of milk and the yoghurt and ginger, and blend to a smooth purée, adding a splash more milk if needed. You could also use a hand blender.

ORCHARD FRUIT OATS

Makes 240ml/8½fl oz (2–3 portions) | ❋ *Suitable for freezing (12 ice cubes)*

Oats are very nutritious and make a great breakfast option. They help to keep energy levels stable and are high in minerals that are essential for healthy bones and teeth.

25g/1oz rolled porridge oats

250ml/9fl oz full-fat milk, plus extra if needed

1 ripe plum, halved, stone removed and the flesh chopped

1 small eating apple, peeled, cored and coarsely grated

1. Soak the oats with the milk and leave overnight, or for a minimum of 1 hour. (While not essential, this speeds up the cooking time and is thought to make them easier to digest.)
2. Tip the oats into a saucepan and stir in the plum and apple. Bring almost to boiling point, then turn down the heat and cook, stirring constantly, for 10 minutes or until the oats are very tender.
3. Mash the mixture until almost smooth, adding a splash more milk if needed. Alternatively, purée in a food processor or using a hand blender – the plum skin takes a little while to break down.

AVOCADO AND SWEET POTATO

Makes 120ml/4½fl oz (1–2 portions)

The avocado gives a lovely creaminess to the sweet potato as well as providing plentiful amounts of heart-friendly nutrients. Make just before serving for the best flavour and colour.

75g/3oz sweet potato, peeled and cut into 1cm/½in chunks

Flesh of ¼ small ripe avocado

2 tbsp full-fat milk (optional)

1. Put the sweet potato in a saucepan then cover with water and bring to the boil. Reduce the heat, cover the pan and simmer for 10–12 minutes or until tender, then drain.
2. Using the back of a fork, mash the sweet potato and avocado until smooth and creamy, adding the milk if the purée is too thick. Alternatively, blend in a food processor or using a hand blender.

TOMATO QUINOA BOWL

Makes 240ml/8½fl oz (2–3 portions) | * *Suitable for freezing (12 ice cubes)*

A healthy start to the day, this savoury 'porridge' is made with protein-rich, energy-sustaining quinoa and egg.

100g/3½oz quinoa

4 tbsp passata

2 tbsp full-fat milk, plus extra if needed

1 hard-boiled egg, peeled and roughly chopped

1. Put the quinoa in a saucepan and cover with water. Bring to the boil, then turn the heat down to low, partially cover the pan and simmer for 15–17 minutes or until the grains are very soft. Cook for slightly longer than usual, so the quinoa is mashable.
2. Drain the quinoa and return it to the pan with the passata and milk, stir well and heat through over a medium-low heat for a couple of minutes.
3. Spoon the quinoa mixture into a bowl and, using the back of a fork, mash in the egg to make a coarse purée. Alternatively, purée in a food processor or using a hand blender, adding a splash more milk if needed.

» There are plenty of vitamins in this dish. Egg is a great source of vitamin D, which keeps our bones, teeth and muscles healthy, and tomatoes contain vitamin C, which is really important for our immune system.

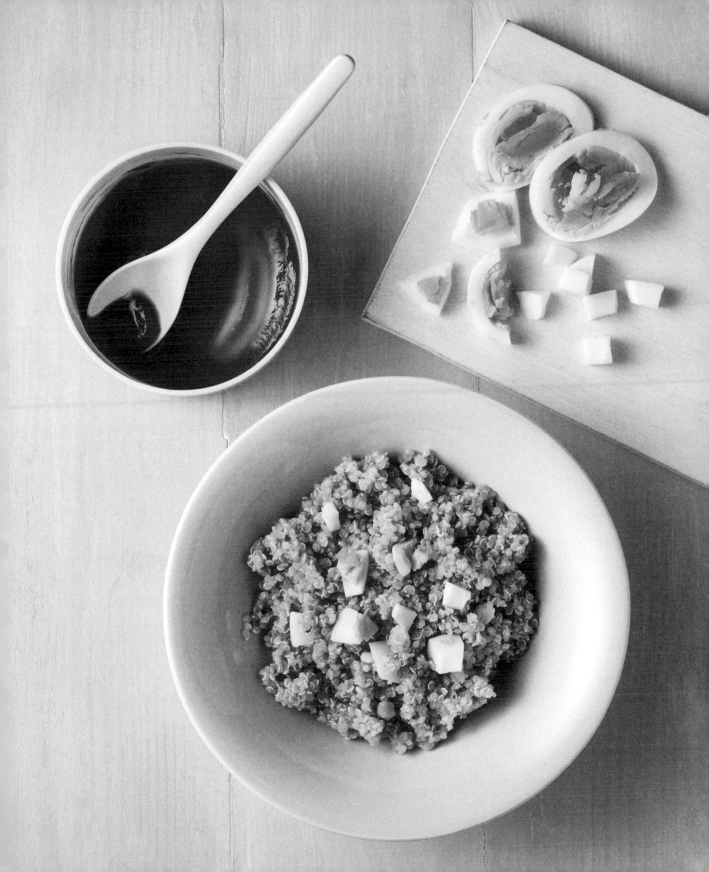

PASTA WITH COURGETTE AND CHEESE

Makes 440ml/15fl oz (4–6 portions) | ❄ *Suitable for freezing (22 ice cubes)*

In Italy, this simple pasta dish is a typical first baby meal. Although often served plain with just butter or olive oil and grated Parmesan, this version also includes courgette. Broccoli, peas, grated cauli, carrots or spinach are other options.

75g/3oz small dried pasta shapes for soup

1 courgette (about 100g/3½oz), finely chopped

8g/⅓oz unsalted butter

8g/⅓oz Parmesan cheese, finely grated

1. Cook the pasta in plenty of unsalted boiling water following the packet instructions.
2. Meanwhile, place the courgette in a saucepan and cover with water. Bring to the boil, then reduce the heat and simmer for 3–5 minutes or until tender. Drain over a bowl, saving 3–4 tablespoons of the cooking water.
3. Put the courgette, butter, cheese and the smaller quantity of saved cooking water in a food processor, or use a hand blender, and purée until smooth.
4. Drain the pasta and combine with the courgette mixture. Mash until almost smooth, adding the rest of the water if needed. Alternatively, blend the pasta with the veg in a food processor or using a hand blender.

BEANS, SWEET POTATO AND CHEESE

Makes 240ml/8½fl oz (2–3 portions) | ❄ *Suitable for freezing (12 ice cubes)*

Potato, beans and cheese are a winning combination. You could make a larger quantity of this purée and serve it for the family as an alternative to regular mash.

115g/4oz sweet potato, peeled and cut into 1cm/½in chunks

60g/2½oz tinned haricot beans, drained and rinsed

8g/⅓oz mature Cheddar cheese, grated

3–4 tbsp full-fat milk

1. Put the sweet potato in a saucepan and cover with water. Bring to the boil, then reduce the heat, cover the pan and simmer for 10–12 minutes. Add the beans and cook for another 3 minutes. Drain and return to the pan, then add the cheese and the smaller quantity of milk and heat through briefly.
2. Using the back of a fork, mash to a coarse purée. Alternatively, purée in a food processor or using a hand blender, adding the remaining milk if needed.

BABY 'BAKED' BEANS

Makes 280ml/10fl oz (2–4 portions) | ❋ *Suitable for freezing (14 ice cubes)*

Not strictly like the kind that comes out of a tin, but these tomatoey beans are no less delicious!

60g/2½oz peeled sweet potato, cut into 1cm/½in chunks

1 carrot (about 50g/2oz), roughly chopped

2 tomatoes, halved and deseeded

75g/3oz tinned haricot beans, drained and rinsed

15g/½oz unsalted butter

3–4 tbsp full-fat milk

1 hard-boiled egg yolk, chopped

1. Put the sweet potato in a saucepan and cover with water. Bring to the boil and cook for 10–12 minutes or until tender.
2. While the sweet potato is cooking, blitz the carrot and tomatoes in a food processor, or using a hand blender, until very finely chopped. Put them in a separate pan with the haricot beans, butter and the smaller quantity of milk and simmer, partially covered with a lid, over a medium-low heat for 10 minutes or until everything is tender and mushy. Stir in the chopped egg yolk.
3. Drain the sweet potato and add to the bean mixture. Using the back of a fork, mash the mixture to a coarse purée, adding the remaining milk if needed. Alternatively, purée in a food processor or using a hand blender.

» Beans are a good source of magnesium, which helps our muscles to work properly.

JAMBALAYA

Makes 120ml/4½fl oz (1–2 portions)

The word 'jambalaya' literally means 'jumbled up' and this mild baby version of the spicy Cajun dish is just that. Don't be put off by the addition of silken tofu. It's rich in protein and is softer and creamier than the regular kind, so blends well with other ingredients. Look for it in the Asian section in large supermarkets or in Asian grocers. You could swap it for the same quantity of cooked chicken or white fish, if you prefer.

15g/½oz white long-grain rice, rinsed

1 tsp olive oil

25g/1oz red pepper (deseeded), diced

1 garlic clove, crushed

2 tsp tomato purée

25g/1oz silken tofu, drained well and grated

Large pinch of mild smoked paprika

3 tbsp almond milk (not rice-based), full-fat cow's milk or boiled water, plus extra if needed

1. Put the rice in a saucepan and cover with water. Bring to the boil, then turn the heat down to low, cover the pan and simmer for 12–15 minutes or until tender.
2. While the rice is cooking, heat the oil in a small pan over a medium-low heat. Add the red pepper and cook for 5 minutes, then add the garlic and cook for another minute. Stir in the tomato purée, tofu, paprika and milk or boiled water and cook for another 5 minutes.
3. Drain the rice and add to the pan with the tofu mixture. Using the back of a fork, mash until almost smooth, adding a splash more milk or boiled water if needed. Alternatively, purée in a food processor or using a hand blender.

SPICED SQUASH, LENTIL AND APPLE

Makes 480ml/17fl oz (4–7 portions) | ❋ *Suitable for freezing (24 ice cubes)*

Gently aromatic rather than hot spices are perfect for introducing your baby to new flavours and widening their palate. Start children early and they're more likely to be unfussy eaters in the future – well, that's the theory!

25g/1oz split red lentils, rinsed

225g/8oz butternut squash, peeled, deseeded and cut into 1cm/½in chunks

1 eating apple, peeled, cored and cut into 1.5cm/⅝in chunks

½ tsp ground coriander

1. Put the lentils in a saucepan, cover with water and bring to the boil. Turn the heat down to low and simmer, partially covered with a lid, for 20 minutes or until tender.

2. While the lentils are cooking, put the squash and apple in a separate pan and cover with water. Bring to the boil, then reduce the heat, cover the pan and simmer for 10–12 minutes or until tender. Drain over a bowl, reserving 4–5 tablespoons of the cooking water.

3. Using the back of a fork, mash the lentils, squash and apple with the ground coriander and the smaller quantity of saved cooking water until almost smooth, adding the remaining water if needed. Alternatively, purée in a food processor or using a hand blender.

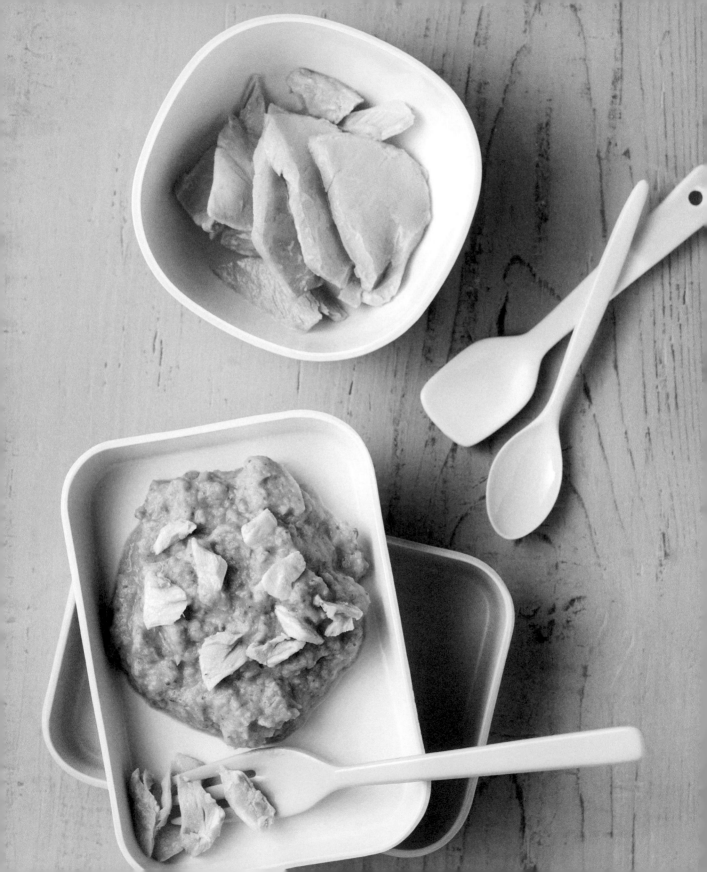

MY FIRST FISH PIE

Makes 280ml/10fl oz (2–4 portions) | ❄ *Suitable for freezing (14 ice cubes)*

A perfect introduction to the numerous health benefits of oily fish, this captures all the elements of a potato-topped fish pie but in a baby-friendly form.

125g/4½ oz sweet potato, peeled and cut into 1cm/½in chunks

2 spring onions, sliced

40g/1½oz small broccoli florets

75g/3oz skinless, boneless salmon fillet

100ml/3½fl oz full-fat milk

1 tbsp full-fat crème fraîche

1. Put the sweet potato in a saucepan and cover with water. Bring to the boil, then reduce the heat, cover the pan and simmer for 7 minutes. Add the spring onions and broccoli, and cook for another 5 minutes or until everything is tender. Drain.

2. Meanwhile, put the salmon in a separate pan, pour over the milk and poach over a gentle heat for 5 minutes or until cooked through. Strain the salmon over a jug and save the milk. Using the back of a fork, mash the fish, taking care to double check for any remaining bones.

3. Drain the sweet potato mixture and add to the milk in the jug, then stir in the crème fraîche and purée using a hand blender, or in a food processor, until almost smooth. Stir in the cooked mashed salmon.

» Oily fish provides omega-3 fatty acids, which support the health of the heart and, as research suggests, also the brain.

SIMPLE SPAGHETTI BOLOGNESE

Makes 480ml/17fl oz (4–7 portions) | ✳ *Suitable for freezing (24 ice cubes)*

Your baby's iron reserves start to diminish at around six months, so it makes sense to regularly provide iron-rich foods, such as beef. For vegetarians, red lentils and other pulses are a good source of the mineral and can be swapped for the beef in this simple spaghetti Bolognese.

1 tsp olive oil

75g/3oz lean beef mince

1 small carrot (about 40g/1½oz), scrubbed/peeled and coarsely grated

1 baby leek (about 40g/1½oz), finely chopped

150ml/5fl oz passata

60ml/2½fl oz Beef Bone Broth (see page 110) or just-boiled water

½ tsp dried oregano

60g/2½oz dried spaghetti

1. Heat the olive oil in a saucepan over a medium heat. Add the mince, carrot and leek, and cook for 5 minutes, stirring frequently, until the meat is browned.
2. Pour in the passata, broth or just-boiled water and add the oregano. Stir well and bring almost to the boil, then turn the heat down to low, cover the pan and cook for 20 minutes, stirring occasionally, until the meat and vegetables are tender.
3. Meanwhile, cook the spaghetti in plenty of unsalted boiling water following the packet instructions. Drain the pasta over a bowl, saving some of the cooking water. Finely chop the pasta and then add it to the meat mixture.
4. Using the back of a fork, mash the pasta mixture until almost smooth, adding a splash of the saved cooking water, if you need to. Alternatively, purée in a food processor or using a hand blender.

PORK AND PEAR

Makes 240ml/8½fl oz (2–3 portions) | ✲ *Suitable for freezing (12 ice cubes)*

Pork is a mild-tasting red meat and is perfect for introducing texture to your baby's meals. When combined with beans, kale and pear, as here, you have a tasty, nutritious meal. If the pear is very ripe, you may not need to cook it; simply mash or blend with the rest of the ingredients before serving.

1 tsp olive oil

75g/3oz lean pork mince

15g/½oz kale leaves, finely chopped

50g/2oz tinned haricot beans, drained and rinsed

1 small ripe pear, peeled, cored and cut into chunks

75ml/3fl oz full-fat milk

1. Heat the oil in a frying pan and fry the mince over a medium-high heat for 5 minutes, stirring frequently, until browned all over. Add the kale, beans and pear, and cook, stirring, for another 5 minutes or until everything is cooked and tender. Add the milk, heat through and remove from the heat.
2. Using the back of a fork, mash the mixture until almost smooth. Alternatively, purée in a food processor or using a hand blender.

WHITE FISH WITH CREAMY CORN

Makes 320ml/11fl oz (2–4 portions) | ✲ *Suitable for freezing (16 ice cubes)*

It's a good idea to familiarize your baby with the flavour of fish, and this is a good starting point, especially since the sweetcorn and milk help to soften any strong fish taste.

125g/4½oz skinless, boneless, thick white fish fillet (e.g. cod or hake), cut into large pieces

60g/2½oz tinned sweetcorn (with no added sugar or salt), drained well

1 tomato, deseeded and roughly chopped

50g/2oz tinned haricot beans, drained and rinsed

1 tsp finely chopped fresh parsley

75ml/3fl oz full-fat milk

Large pinch of ground turmeric

1. Put the fish, sweetcorn, tomato, beans, parsley and milk in a saucepan. Cook, covered with a lid, over a medium-low heat for 5–7 minutes or until the fish is cooked through. Check for any bones, then stir in the turmeric.
2. Using the back of a fork, mash the mixture until almost smooth. Alternatively, purée in a food processor or using a hand blender.

EASY CHICKEN TAGINE

Makes 480ml/17fl oz (4–7 portions) | * *Suitable for freezing (24 ice cubes)*

Don't feel you have to stick to mild-tasting meals for your child; many babies like stronger flavours, especially if they are breastfed and have experienced these through your breast milk. Aromatic, rather than hot, spices, including nutmeg, cinnamon, mixed spice, cumin and coriander, will add interest to their meals and expand their palate, though just keep it to a pinch for now.

1 tsp olive oil

½ onion, finely chopped

150g/5oz butternut squash, peeled, deseeded and cut into 1cm/½in chunks

100g/3½oz skinless, boneless chicken breast, cut into1cm/½in chunks

1 unsulphured dark dried apricot, chopped

50g/2oz tinned chickpeas, drained and rinsed

150ml/5fl oz Chicken Bone Broth (see page 111) or just-boiled water

Large pinch each of ground cinnamon and ground coriander

1. Heat the oil in a saucepan, add the onion and squash, and cook over a medium heat for 5 minutes or until softened, stirring frequently and adding a splash of water if needed.
2. Stir in the chicken, apricot and chickpeas, and cook for another 5 minutes. Pour in the broth or just-boiled water and stir in the spices. Cook over a low heat for 10 minutes, partially covered with a lid and stirring frequently, until reduced.
3. Using the back of a fork, mash the mixture until almost smooth. Alternatively, purée in a food processor or using a hand blender.

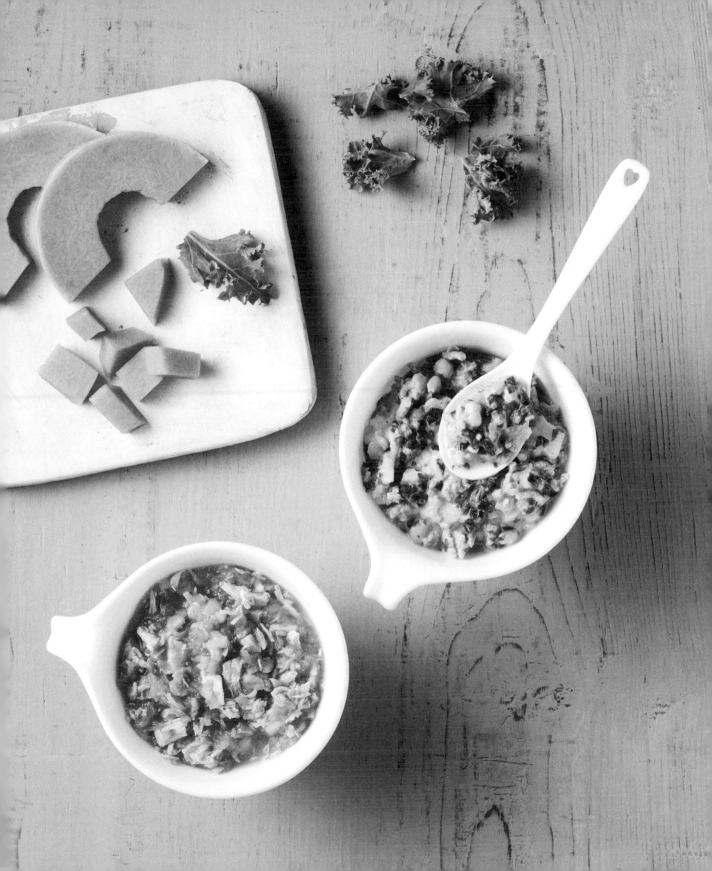

LAMB AND APRICOT COUSCOUS

Makes 240ml/8½fl oz (2–3 portions) | ❋ *Suitable for freezing (12 ice cubes)*

Look for dark dried apricots, rather than the bright orange ones, to make this tagine-style recipe. Not only do they taste better but they are a great source of potassium, which is needed to keep our nervous systems healthy and our muscles functioning properly. Check the packet to make sure they come without the preservative sulphur, which it is thought might aggravate asthma symptoms in susceptible children and adults.

25g/1oz couscous

125g/4½oz butternut squash, peeled, deseeded and cut into 1cm/½in chunks

2 unsulphured dark dried apricots, chopped

1 tsp olive oil

1 tbsp finely chopped onion

75g/3oz lean lamb mince

Large pinch of ground ginger (optional)

1. Put the couscous in a bowl and pour over enough just-boiled water to cover. Give the couscous a stir, then cover with a plate and leave until ready to use.
2. Put the squash in a saucepan, cover with water and bring to the boil. Turn the heat down slightly, cover the pan and simmer for 10–12 minutes or until the squash is tender, adding the apricots after 5 minutes.
3. While the squash is cooking, heat the olive oil in a frying pan, add the onion and mince, and cook over a medium heat, stirring, for 10 minutes until the lamb is browned and cooked through. Stir in the ginger, if using.
4. Drain the squash and apricots over a bowl, saving 2–3 tablespoons of the cooking water. Tip the squash and apricots into the frying pan, along with the couscous and the smaller quantity of saved water, and mash to a coarse purée with the back of a fork, adding the remaining water if needed. Alternatively, purée in a food processor or using a hand blender.

CHICKEN MINESTRONE

Makes 480ml/17fl oz (4–7 portions) | ❊ *Suitable for freezing (24 ice cubes)*

Fennel seeds may seem a bit unusual for babies but they are a traditional remedy for digestion that has long been believed to help ease trapped wind. They do have a distinctive flavour, however, so can be left out if your baby finds them too strong. Orzo may look like grains of rice, but it's actually a type of pasta and is the perfect size for little ones.

75g/3oz dried orzo pasta

2 tsp olive oil

1 baby leek (about 40g/1½oz), finely chopped

15g/½oz baby leaf spinach, finely chopped

2 tomatoes, deseeded and diced

200ml/7fl oz Chicken Bone Broth (see page 111) or just-boiled water, plus extra if needed

Pinch of ground fennel seeds (optional)

50g/2oz cooked chicken, finely chopped

1. Cook the orzo in plenty of unsalted boiling water following the packet instructions, then drain.
2. While the pasta is cooking, heat the oil in a saucepan over a medium-low heat. Add the leek, spinach and tomatoes, and cook for 3 minutes, stirring.
3. Pour in the broth or just-boiled water and add the fennel seeds, if using. Cook, partially covered with a lid, for another 3 minutes, then add the chicken and heat through. Stir in the cooked pasta.
4. Using the back of a fork, mash until almost smooth, adding a splash more broth or boiled water if needed. Alternatively, purée in a food processor or using a hand blender.

CHERRY, CARROT AND YOGHURT

Makes 160ml/5½fl oz (1–2 portions) | ❄ *Suitable for freezing (8 ice cubes)*

A bag of black cherries is a great asset in the freezer – especially as they come pitted so there's no fiddly preparation. Carrots are high in vitamin A, which supports the immune system and helps to keep the skin and eyes healthy. In natural medicine, cherries are said to help promote sleep – a win-win for me.

1 carrot (about 50g/2oz), scrubbed/peeled and diced

100g/3½oz frozen pitted black cherries

2 tbsp thick plain full-fat live yoghurt, plus extra if needed

1. Put the carrot in a small saucepan, cover with water and bring to the boil. Turn the heat down slightly and cook for 5 minutes. Add the cherries and cook for another 3 minutes or until the carrot is tender and the cherries warmed through and defrosted.
2. Drain the carrot and cherries, and tip them into a jug with the yoghurt. Purée in a food processor or using a hand blender until smooth, adding more yoghurt, if needed.

TROPICAL RICE PUDDING

Makes 240ml/8½fl oz (2–3 portions)

Mango and coconut give an interesting twist to classic rice pudding. Although coconut isn't strictly a nut, do be mindful of giving it to your baby if there's any history of nut and seed allergies. You could make this with cow's milk and omit the desiccated coconut, if you prefer.

25g/1oz white long-grain rice, rinsed

75g/3oz ripe mango flesh, cut into chunks

1 tsp desiccated coconut

3 tbsp coconut drinking milk (from a carton), plus extra if needed

Large pinch of nutmeg (optional)

1. Put the rice in a small saucepan and cover with water. Bring to the boil, then turn the heat down to low, cover the pan and simmer for 12 minutes until almost cooked.
2. Add the mango and desiccated coconut, and cook for another 3 minutes. Drain and return the rice mixture to the pan with the coconut milk and nutmeg, if using.
3. Using the back of a fork, mash the mixture until almost smooth, adding more milk, if needed. Alternatively, purée in a food processor or using a hand blender.

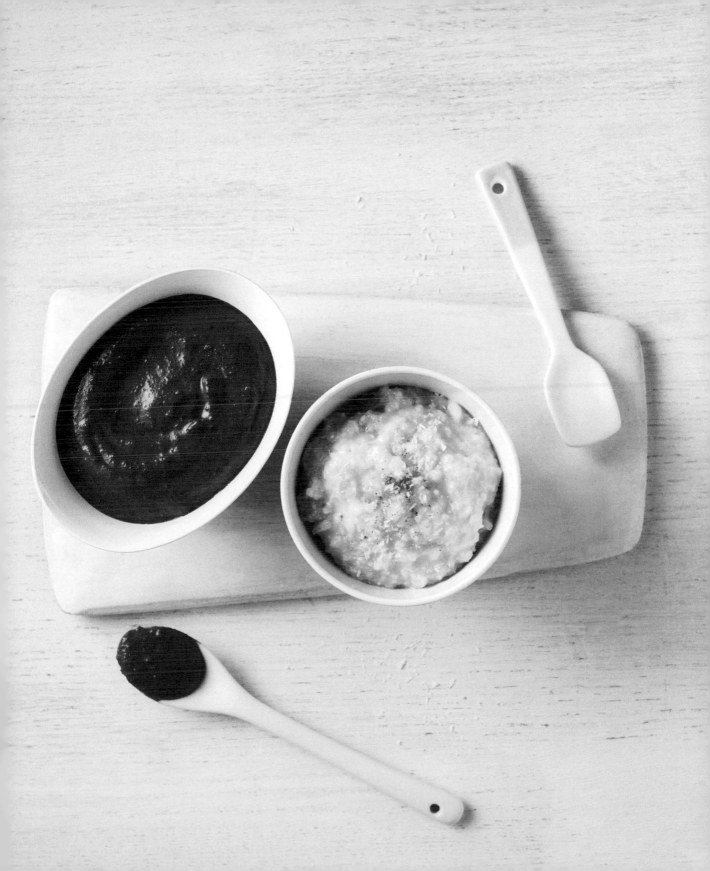

AVOCADO AND MANGO

Makes 125ml/4½fl oz (1–2 portions)

This makes a lovely creamy, filling purée with bountiful amounts of nutrients and healthy fats.

Flesh of ½ small ripe avocado, chopped

Squeeze of lemon juice

25g/1oz ripe mango flesh, chopped

1 tbsp plain full-fat live Greek yoghurt

Using the back of a fork, mash all the ingredients until smooth. Alternatively, purée in a food processor or using a hand blender.

PEACH AND COTTAGE CHEESE

Makes 125ml/4½fl oz (1–2 portions)

Mild-tasting and high in protein and calcium, cottage cheese is good for your baby's growing bones. As cottage cheese is often considered a diet food, it's important to go for a full-fat version, rather than a low-fat one. Health experts recommend that babies and young children should not be given low-fat food until two years of age, at which point it can be gradually introduced, as long as they are eating well. It is also worth noting that children under the age of five shouldn't be given skimmed milk as a drink as it doesn't provide the energy and contain the vitamin A they need at this stage.

1 ripe peach

3 tbsp full-fat cottage cheese

1. If you want to remove the skin, place the peach in a bowl and pour over enough just-boiled water from a kettle to cover. Leave for 30 seconds, then scoop up the peach using a slotted spoon and cool briefly under cold running water. Peel off the skin, cut the fruit in half and remove the stone.
2. Using the back of a fork, mash the peach with the cottage cheese in a bowl to a coarse purée. Alternatively, purée in a food processor or using a hand blender.

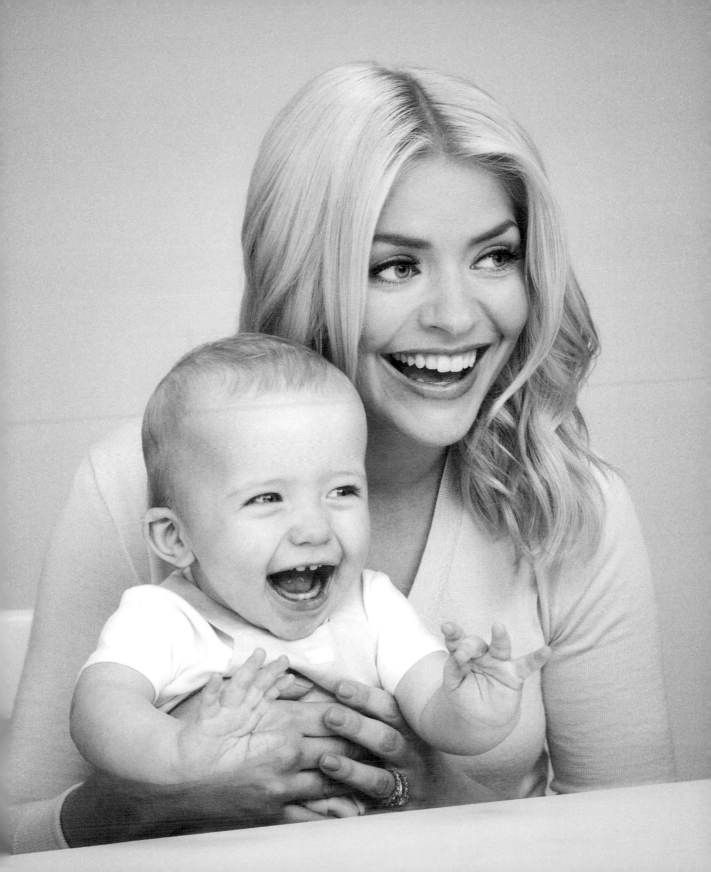

PEAR AND BLUEBERRY

Makes 160ml/5½fl oz (1–2 portions) | ❋ *Suitable for freezing (8 ice cubes)*

You do need a juicy ripe pear for this quick, no-fuss purée. It would also make a delicious smoothie blended with full-fat, thick, plain live yoghurt, full-fat milk and a splash of vanilla extract – yum!

1 small ripe pear, peeled, cored and chopped

50g/2oz blueberries

Using the back of a fork, mash the pear and blueberries to make a smooth – or smoothish – purée. You can press the mixture through a sieve to get rid of the blueberry skins, if you prefer. Alternatively, purée using a food processor or hand blender.

MELON AND COTTAGE CHEESE

Makes 125ml/4½fl oz (1–2 portions)

This is perfect for when time is short. No cooking is needed and it takes mere minutes to rustle up.

60g/2½oz ripe honeydew melon flesh, chopped

60g/2½oz full-fat cottage cheese

¼ tsp ground flaxseeds/linseeds (optional)

Using the back of a fork, mash the melon and cottage cheese in a bowl to a coarse purée, then stir in the ground flaxseeds (if using). Alternatively, purée in a food processor or using a hand blender.

VEGETABLE STOCK

Makes about 1 litre/1¾ pints | ❄ *Suitable for freezing*

Making your own stock is pretty easy and you can rest assured that it's free from additives or salt. This light, flavoursome stock makes a great drink or can be used as a base for soups, sauces and stews. Feel free to swap the veg for any you have in the kitchen, but avoid using too much of one type as its flavour could be too overpowering.

1 tbsp olive oil

2 onions, chopped

2 large leeks, chopped

4 carrots, scrubbed/peeled and chopped

2 celery sticks, sliced

1 potato (about 250g/9oz), peeled and quartered

3 garlic cloves, peeled and left whole

1 handful of fresh parsley (leaves and stalks)

2 bay leaves

½ tsp whole black peppercorns

1. Heat the olive oil in a large saucepan over a medium heat, add the onions and cook, stirring frequently, for 5 minutes. Add the rest of the vegetables and the garlic, and cook for another 5 minutes.
2. Pour in 1.5 litres/2½ pints of water, or enough to cover the vegetables, and stir in the parsley, bay leaves and peppercorns. Bring to the boil, then turn the heat down to a simmer, cover with a lid and cook for 40 minutes. Remove from the heat and leave to cool. Strain the stock into a large bowl in batches, picking out the peppercorns and bay leaves as you go.
3. Leave to cool and then store in a sterilized airtight container in the fridge for up to a week, or freeze in portions. Don't discard the cooked vegetables but blend them into a delicious purée or, with added stock, into a nutritious thick broth.

BEEF BONE BROTH

Makes about 1.5 litres/2½ pints | ❄ *Suitable for freezing*

This is a bit of a labour of love but you'll be blessed for your patience with a nourishing, flavoursome no-salt broth. Research has shown that, due to the high gelatine and collagen content of bone broth, it has some anti-inflammatory qualities. It is also believed to help improve the health of the lining of the gut, as well as promoting healthy bones, skin, hair and nails. The broth can be made in bulk, frozen in portions and used as a base for sauces, soups and stews. Ask your butcher for organic bones, preferably from grass-fed cows.

2kg/4lb 6oz organic beef bones

1 large onion, cut into wedges

2 carrots, scrubbed/peeled and thickly sliced

1 garlic bulb (unpeeled), cut in half

1 celery stick, thickly sliced

5 whole black peppercorns

1. First, blanch the bones to remove any impurities. Place in a large saucepan, cover with water and bring to the boil over a high heat. Turn the heat down slightly, partially cover with a lid and cook at a rolling boil for 25 minutes before draining.

2. Next roast the bones in the oven, which will give the stock a rich beefy flavour. Preheat the oven to 240°C/475°F/Gas 9. Spread out the drained bones in two baking trays and roast for 30 minutes until browned and caramelized.

3. Return the bones to the large pan, add the onion, carrots, garlic, celery and peppercorns, and pour in enough water to cover – about 2 litres/3½ pints. Bring to the boil, then turn the heat down to low, cover the pan and simmer for 8–12 hours; the longer you cook it, the better the flavour will be. Keep an eye on the water level and top up occasionally, if you need to.

4. When the broth is ready, lift out the bones using tongs and discard, then strain through a sieve into a bowl, pressing the vegetables through the sieve with the back of a spoon. Discard the peppercorns, and any other remnants left in the sieve. The broth is ready to use straight away (to intensify its flavour return it to the pan and cook until reduced by a third).

5. Alternatively, leave the broth to cool, scoop off any fat on the surface and store in a sterilized airtight container in the fridge for up to three days, or divide into portions and keep in the freezer for up to three months.

CHICKEN BONE BROTH

Makes about 1.5 litres/2½ pints | ❋ *Suitable for freezing*

Shop-bought stocks are often laden with salt and additives, so it really makes sense to make your own. You'll be rewarded with a flavoursome broth that is also beneficial to the health of your baby (see Beef Bone Broth on page 110). The easiest, most economical and waste-free way to make this is to use the chicken carcass from a roast, or to strip the meat from a whole cooked chicken.

1 leftover chicken carcass from a roast

1 large onion, cut into wedges

2 carrots, scrubbed/peeled and thickly sliced

1 garlic bulb (unpeeled), cut in half

1 celery stick, thickly sliced

5 whole black peppercorns

1. Put the chicken carcass in a large saucepan and cover with water. Add the onion, carrots, garlic, celery and peppercorns, and pour in enough water to cover – about 2 litres/3½ pints. Bring to the boil, then turn the heat down to low, cover the pan and simmer for 2 hours. Keep an eye on the water level and top up occasionally, if you need to.

2. Lift out the chicken carcass using tongs and discard, then strain the broth through a sieve into a bowl, pressing the vegetables through the sieve with the back of a spoon. Discard the peppercorns and any other remnants left in the sieve. The broth is ready to use straight away (to intensify its flavour return it to the pan and cook until reduced by a third).

3. Leave the broth to cool, scoop off any fat on the surface and store in a sterilized airtight container in the fridge for up to three days, or divide into portions and keep in the freezer for up to three months.

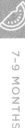

7–9 MONTHS

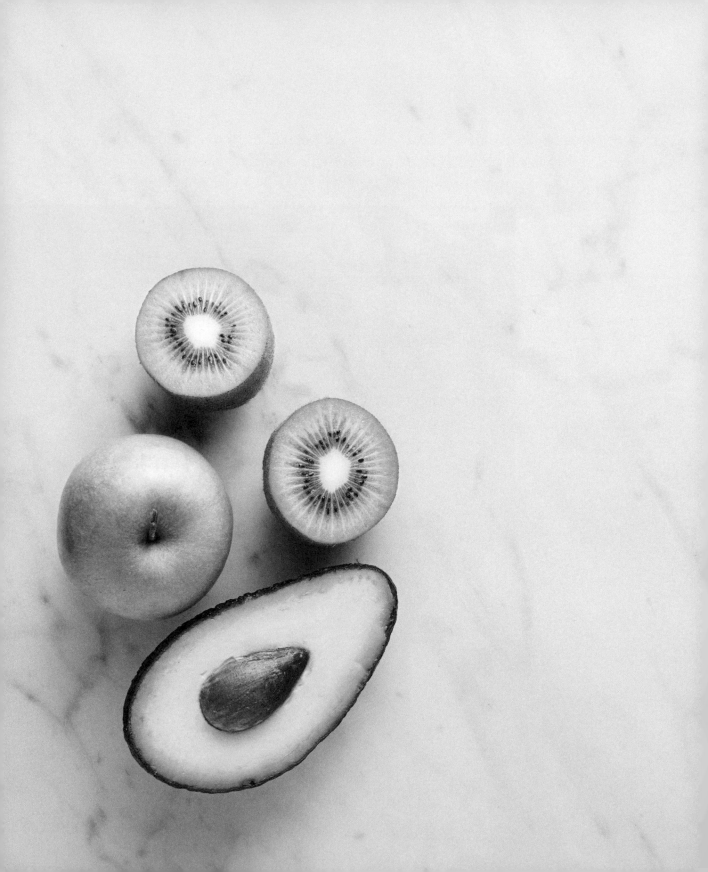

Chapter 3

9–12 MONTHS

Food is now very interesting to your baby and in the three months leading up to his first birthday he will hopefully be starting to tuck into three meals a day. Ideally, you'll find yourself preparing baby-specific meals less and less. You'll find quite a few recipes in this chapter that are suitable for the whole family, although you should always remove your little one's portion before seasoning the rest of the dish to your taste.

He'll be starting to realize that food is an important part of his daily routine. You might begin to notice that he is beginning to have favourite and not-so-favourite foods, although the same advice applies as ever: persist with the foods that your baby doesn't immediately take to!

HOW MUCH TO FEED YOUR BABY

Once again, I'm keen to remind you that all babies are different, so they'll likely be eating different amounts at mealtimes. Very broadly, I'd say aim for one baby bowl(ish) portion per meal, with some finger food on the side so they keep developing that all-important pincer grip.

No matter what stage your baby is at physically, he'll be on the move in some capacity, be it crawling, pulling himself up or walking. Make sure his meals contain foods that are packed with energy-rich nutrients to fuel all his new antics. Beans and pulses are particularly great for little movers! I liked to start mine off with Baby Granola Sprinkle (see page 118), which is packed with oats, nuts and seeds, or Smoky Beans and Egg (see page 121), which has plenty of protein to keep your little one going.

Aside from around three main meals each day, he might also need a few small snacks for an extra energy boost. Hopefully he'll be getting more adept with his new-found pincer grip – in which case, veggie and fruit sticks make great snacks. You'll also find some fun ideas in the Baby-led Weaning chapter (see pages 180–207). Chester and Belle loved dunking Baked Falafel Balls in Roasted Red Pepper Dip (see pages 202 and 201). And Frozen Banana Pops (see page 206) were great snacks for when my little ones were teething, although take care not to let your baby get too full on these before a meal and, to be on the safe side, never leave him alone with finger foods.

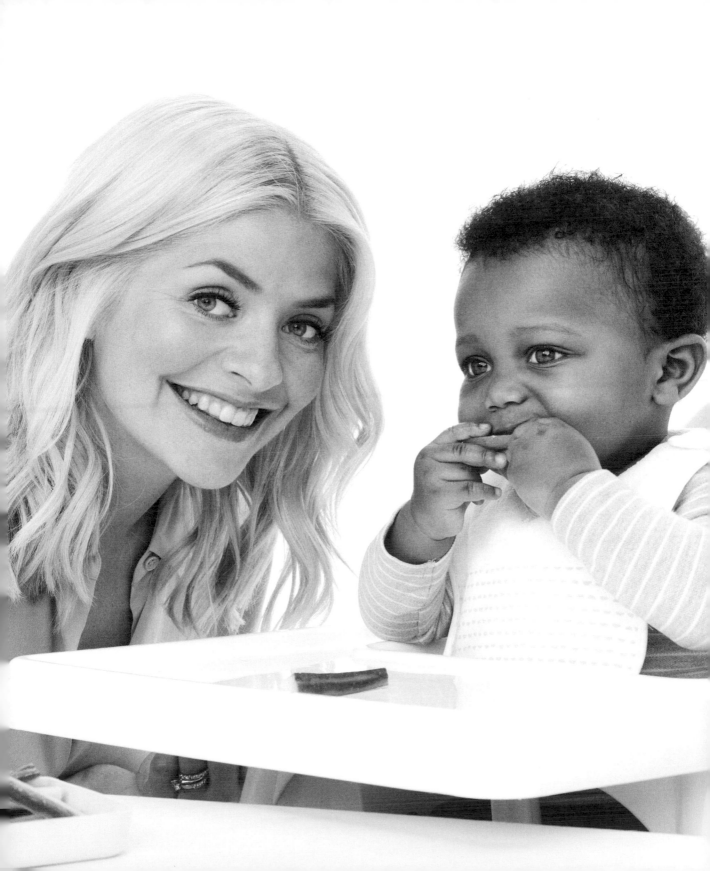

TEXTURE

By the end nine months, you should be offering lumpier foods – no more smooth purées! Minced or chopped foods with lumps are what's required now, so your baby can really get to grips with chewing and swallowing. At this stage, mine particularly took to Veggie Scramble, with slightly chunkier bits of avocado in it (see page 121).

BREASTFEEDING/MILK

As your baby begins to eat more meals and thicker textures, you'll find he might naturally start to show less interest in milk feeds. With all of mine, the late-night feed was the first to go, followed by the mid-morning feed, then eventually the mid-afternoon feed. Your baby still needs milk, though, so keep up the waking and before-bed feeds that, combined with the milk incorporated in cooking, should be enough to ensure they're still having the minimum 400–600ml/14fl oz–1 pint intake required for babies under a year old.

SAMPLE MENU

🕐 **Breakfast**

Smoky Beans and Egg (see page 121) and half a pear, peeled and cut into pieces

🕐 **Mid-morning**

Baby's usual milk feed

🕐 **Lunch**

Well-cooked pasta shapes mixed with some Super-veg Green Pesto (see page 124) and with a few cooked carrot sticks on the side

🕐 **Mid-afternoon**

Baby's usual milk feed, and a Swirly Strawberry Cashew Pot (see page118) as a snack

🕐 **Teatime**

Perhaps try Oven-baked Fish with Squash (see page 127), or Pea and Mint Risotto (see page 122) if you are vegetarian. Try including some soft finger foods, too, such as cooked broccoli florets or fine green beans, and follow with a few pieces of fresh fruit

🕐 **Bedtime**

Baby's usual milk feed

BABY GRANOLA SPRINKLE

Makes 75g/3oz

A sprinkling of this oat, nut and seed granola gives a nutritional boost to yoghurt, fruit sauces and shop-bought cereals. You could even stir it into a fruit-crumble topping. Make sure you blitz the granola into fine crumbs to avoid any risk of choking.

25g/1oz jumbo porridge oats

25g/1oz sunflower seeds

25g/1oz flaked almonds

¼ tsp ground cinnamon

1. Put the oats, seeds and flaked almonds in a large frying pan and toast over a medium-low heat for 2 minutes, tossing the pan occasionally, until just starting to turn golden.
2. Tip the oat mixture into a spice/coffee grinder or food processor, add the cinnamon and blitz very finely. Store in an airtight jar or container for up to two weeks.

SWIRLY STRAWBERRY CASHEW POT

Serves 2–3 (babies/young children)

Cashew nuts make a surprisingly creamy purée when soaked and blended. They are also rich in minerals, including magnesium, zinc and iron.

60g/2½oz cashew nuts

2 soft pitted dates, chopped

100g/3½oz strawberries, hulled and chopped

½ tsp vanilla extract

¼ tsp ground cinnamon

1. Put the cashews and dates in a small bowl, pour over just enough water to cover and leave to soak for at least 1 hour, or overnight if you have time.
2. Drain the cashews and dates, and tip them into a food processor or blender with 3 tablespoons of boiled water from a kettle. Add the rest of the ingredients, setting aside a third of the strawberries, and blend until smooth and creamy – scrape down the sides of the processor/blender so that everything is evenly mixed.
3. Use the back of a fork to mash the reserved strawberries, or blend in the food processor, then stir them gently into the cashew cream to make a swirly pattern. Spoon into ramekins or small bowls to serve or store in the fridge for up to two days.

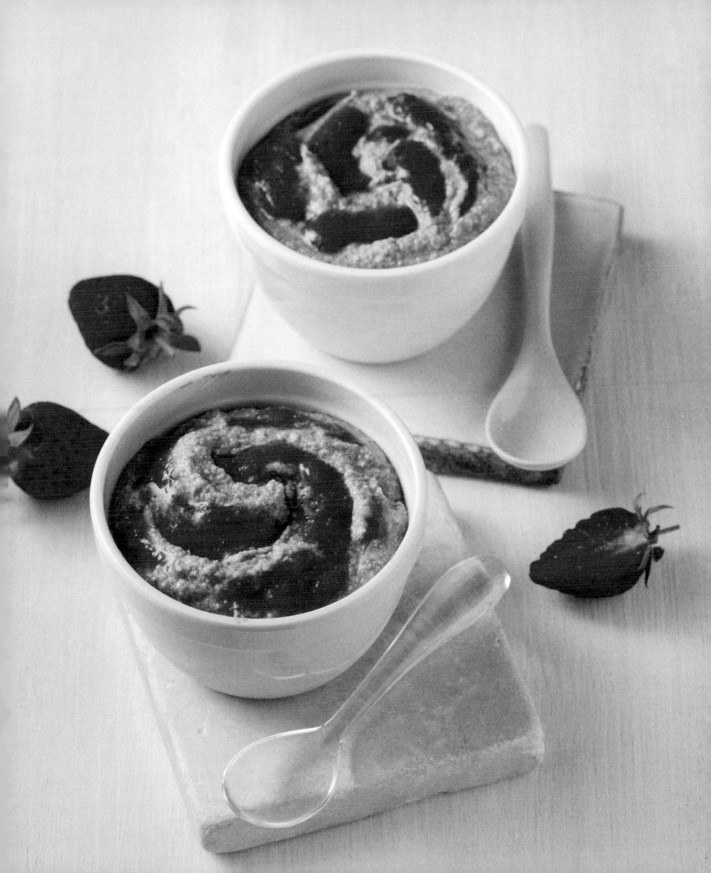

HOTCAKE DUNKERS WITH FRUITY YOGHURT DIP

Makes about 16 pancakes | ❈ *Suitable for freezing (pancakes only)*

Babies love the feeling of independence that comes from eating with their fingers, and these small pancakes are perfect. They taste delicious dunked into this fruity yoghurt dip – you may need to turn a blind eye to the mess!

25g/1oz soft pitted dates, chopped

50g/2oz full-fat cottage cheese

100ml/3½fl oz full-fat milk

1 egg

100g/3½oz self-raising flour

½ tsp ground cinnamon

Unsalted butter or sunflower oil, for cooking

For the fruity yoghurt dip

1 quantity of Pear and Blueberry purée (see page 108)

6 tbsp thick plain full-fat live yoghurt

1. Put the dates in a small bowl and cover with 2 tablespoons of just-boiled water from a kettle. Leave to soften for 15 minutes, then place the dates and their soaking water in a blender with the cottage cheese, milk and egg, and blend until smooth. Pour into a jug.
2. Sift together the flour and cinnamon, and gradually whisk in the date mixture to make a smooth, thick batter. Leave to rest for 20 minutes.
3. Heat enough butter or oil to coat the base of a large frying pan. Place 2 tablespoons of the batter in the pan per pancake and repeat to make four pancakes, then cook each pancake over a medium heat for about 2 minutes on each side or until golden.
4. Keep the pancakes warm in a low oven while you make all 16 pancakes. Mix the Pear and Blueberry purée into the yoghurt in a small bowl or bowls and serve with the pancakes for dunking.

» It's important to include finger foods in your little one's diet as these help your child to strengthen his pincer grip, while chewing more solid foods helps develop the jaw muscles for speech.

SMOKY BEANS AND EGG

Serves 2 (babies/young children) | ❋ *Suitable for freezing*

It's so easy to make baked beans, and these have a slightly smoky-bacon flavour thanks to the smoked paprika. Brillant with toast fingers for dunking.

100g/3½oz tinned haricot beans, drained and rinsed

Large pinch of mild smoked paprika

2 tomatoes, deseeded and roughly chopped

2 tsp tomato purée

15g/½oz unsalted butter

6 tbsp full-fat milk, plus extra if needed

1 hard-boiled egg, peeled and chopped

1. Put the beans, paprika, tomatoes, tomato purée, butter and milk in a small saucepan and cook over a medium-low heat, stirring frequently, for 5 minutes or until the beans are very tender. Stir in the egg.
2. Using the back of a fork, mash to a coarse purée, adding a splash more milk if needed. Alternatively, finely chop.

VEGGIE SCRAMBLE

Serves 2 (babies/young children)

Eggs are a true superfood, containing loads of the essential micronutrients a baby needs, but cook them well, making sure the white and yolk are set.

15g/½oz unsalted butter

1 tomato, deseeded and diced

2 eggs, lightly beaten

2 tbsp full-fat milk

Flesh of ½ small ripe avocado, diced

Freshly ground black pepper

1 small pitta bread, warmed and cut into fingers, to serve

1. Heat half the butter in a small saucepan over a medium-low heat and cook the tomato for 3 minutes, stirring frequently, until softened.
2. Whisk together the eggs and milk in a bowl or jug, seasoning with a grind of black pepper.
3. Melt the remaining butter in the pan and pour in the egg mixture. Cook over a low heat, stirring and folding the eggs continuously for 3–4 minutes or until scrambled and well cooked.
4. Roughly mash in the avocado using the back of a fork. Serve with fingers of pitta bread.

PEA AND MINT RISOTTO

Serves 3 (babies/young children)

Soft and creamy risotto rice is the perfect comfort food for your baby, though you could use the same quantity of white long-grain rice (or half white/half brown) for convenience instead. The pea, leek and mint purée adds a great colour and flavour to the mild-tasting rice and could even be served on its own, or as a side with chicken, fish, pork or lamb. A small amount of cheese is included here, but take care not to give too much to babies under the age of one as it can be high in salt.

75g/3oz risotto rice

100g/3½oz frozen peas

2 baby leeks, sliced

1 tbsp finely chopped fresh
  mint leaves

5g/¼oz unsalted butter

20g/¾oz Parmesan cheese,
  finely grated

1. Put the rice in a saucepan, cover with water and bring to the boil. Turn the heat down to low and simmer, stirring frequently, for 15–18 minutes or until the grains of rice are tender and creamy.
2. While the rice is cooking, place the peas and leeks in a separate pan, cover with water and bring to the boil. Turn down the heat, cover the pan and simmer for about 5 minutes or until tender, then drain. Tip the vegetables and mint into a food processor, or use a hand blender, and blitz to a purée.
3. Drain the rice and return it to the pan, then add the butter, most of the Parmesan and vegetable purée, and stir until combined. Using the back of a fork, mash the risotto to a creamy consistency then sprinkle over the remaining Parmesan.

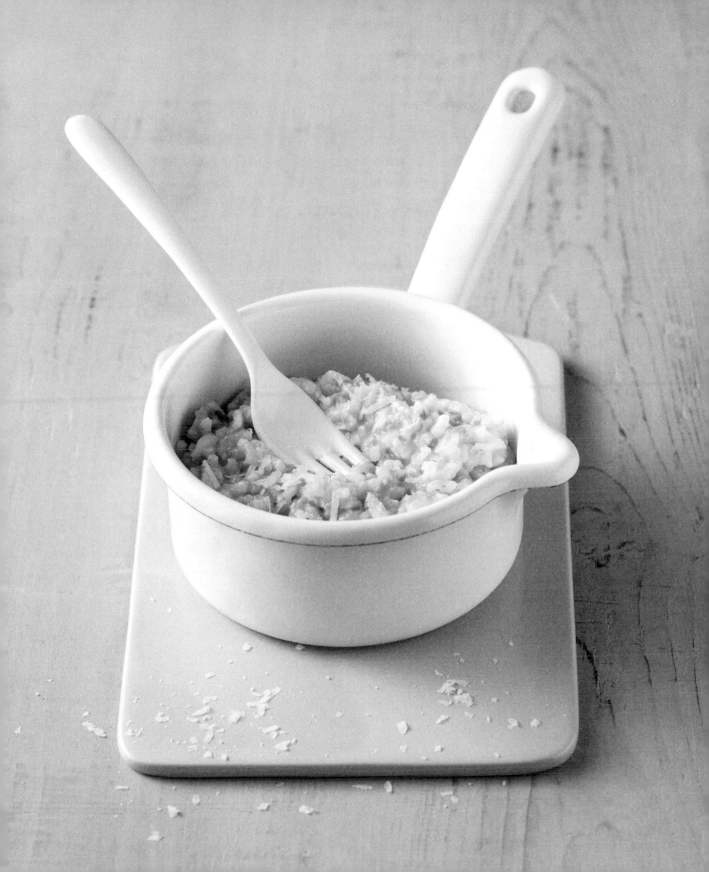

SUPER-VEG GREEN PESTO

Serves about 10 (babies/young children)

This vibrant fresh green sauce looks like regular pesto but is boosted with kale and broccoli. It's a great way of encouraging young kids to eat greens as the extra veg are virtually undetectable. The sauce is well worth storing in a jar in the fridge – it will keep for 1–2 weeks – for when you want to rustle up a quick pesto pasta or stir a spoonful into rice, mash, couscous or quinoa.

1 large garlic clove, peeled and cut in half

100ml/3½fl oz extra-virgin olive oil

25g/1oz cashew nuts

15g/½oz kale leaves

50g/2oz broccoli florets

20g/¾oz fresh basil leaves

25g/1oz Parmesan cheese, finely grated

1. To soften the strong flavour of the raw garlic, put it in a small saucepan with the olive oil and warm gently for 2 minutes, then leave it to cool in the oil.
2. Meanwhile, put the cashews in a food processor or a spice/coffee grinder and process until very finely chopped. Tip the chopped nuts into a bowl.
3. Using a slotted spoon, fish out the garlic from the oil in the saucepan and put it in the food processor, along with the kale, broccoli and basil, and blitz until very finely chopped.
4. Spoon the vegetable mixture into the bowl with the chopped nuts. Stir in the Parmesan and the garlic-infused olive oil from the pan until mixed together. Use straight away or spoon the pesto into a sterilized jar and store, covered, in the fridge until ready to use.

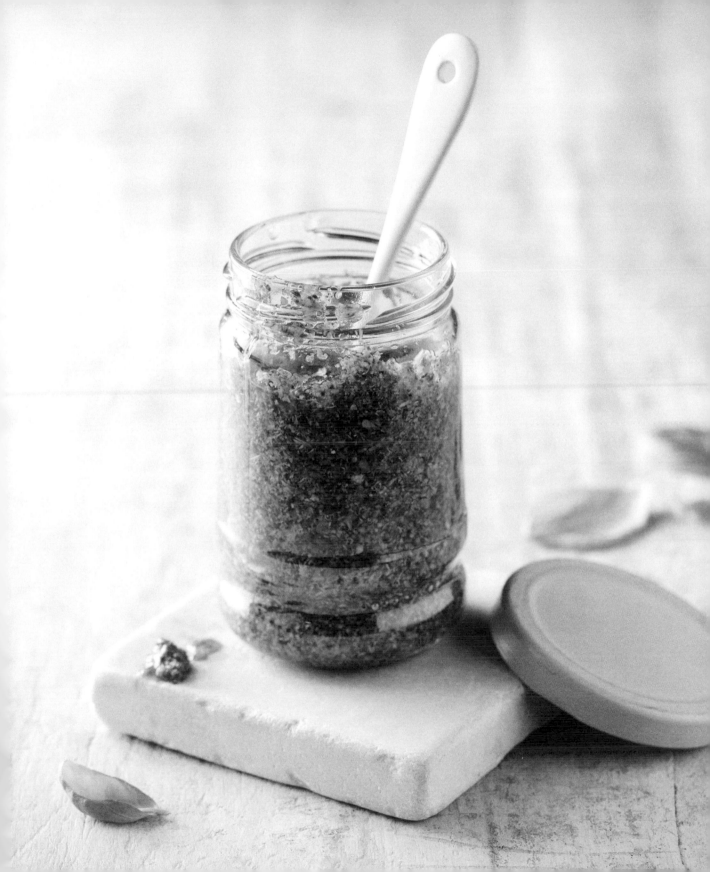

COCONUT FISH WITH QUINOA

Serves 2–3 (babies/young children) | ❆ *Suitable for freezing*

Don't discount quinoa as just the 'trendy' grain of the moment – it has a lot going for it: it's the perfect size for babies, it is easy to cook and offers many health benefits.

40g/1½oz quinoa

1 tsp coconut oil or sunflower oil

1 small leek, finely chopped

¼ tsp grated fresh root ginger

¼–½ tsp mild curry powder

100ml/3½fl oz coconut drinking milk (from a carton), plus extra if needed

25g/1oz frozen peas

125g/4½oz skinless, boneless thick white fish fillet, flesh cut into small bite-sized pieces

1. Put the quinoa in a saucepan, cover with water and bring to the boil. Turn the heat down to low, cover the pan and simmer for 15–17 minutes (cook it for slightly longer than usual so the grains are very soft).

2. While the quinoa is cooking, heat the oil in a small pan and add the leek and ginger. Cook for 5 minutes until softened before stirring in the curry powder, coconut milk and peas. Cook for another 5 minutes until the vegetables are tender.

3. Double check the fish for any bones, then stir it into the leek mixture in the pan and cook for 3 minutes or until cooked through and flaky.

4. Using the back of a fork, mash the fish mixture to a coarse purée. Stir in the quinoa and mash again, if needed. Add a splash more coconut milk if the mixture is too thick.

» Quinoa is a complete form of protein, offering all nine essential amino acids – rare for a plant-based protein – and it is also a good source of iron and magnesium.

OVEN-BAKED FISH WITH SQUASH

Serves 2–3 (babies/young children) | ❄ *Suitable for freezing*

Super-easy – the fish is baked in a foil parcel at the same time as the squash is roasting, so there's no need for lots of pans or washing-up! It's one of those recipes that can easily be doubled, or made to serve more, depending on the number of people you are feeding.

100g/3½ oz butternut squash, peeled, deseeded and cut into 1cm/½in chunks

1 tsp olive oil, plus extra for drizzling

1 small leek, finely chopped

125g/4½oz skinless, boneless thick white fish fillet

2 tomatoes, deseeded and chopped

1 tsp chopped fresh parsley

Squeeze of lemon juice

1. Preheat the oven to 180°C/350°F/Gas 4.
2. Put the butternut squash in a bowl, pour over the olive oil and toss with your hands until the squash is coated all over. Tip the squash on to a baking tray, spreading it out evenly and leaving a space in the middle for the fish parcel, then roast in the oven for 10 minutes.
3. Meanwhile, tear off a sheet of foil large enough to make a parcel to hold the fish. Scatter the leek in the middle of the foil and top with the fish, tomatoes and parsley. Add a squeeze of lemon juice and drizzle over a little olive oil.
4. Seal the foil parcel, tucking in the edges. Remove the tray from the oven, add the parcel and cook in the oven for 20 minutes or until the fish is cooked, the leeks are soft and the squash is tender but not crisp.
5. Put the roasted squash in a bowl. Open the foil parcel and add the contents to the bowl. Using the back of a fork, mash to a coarse purée. Alternatively, finely chop.

SUNNY SALMON AND CORN CHOWDER

Serves 2–3 (babies/young children) | ✳ *Suitable for freezing*

The turmeric not only gives this fish chowder a lovely golden colour but it's good for the health of your baby, too. Research has shown that it has both anti-inflammatory and antioxidant properties, which are enhanced by combining it with a little black pepper.

125g/4oz new potatoes (such as Charlotte; unpeeled), cut into 1cm/½in chunks

1 carrot (about 60g/2½oz), scrubbed/peeled and cut into chunks

75g/3oz skinless, boneless salmon fillet, flesh cut into small bite-sized pieces

125ml/4½fl oz full-fat milk, plus extra if needed

4 tbsp tinned sweetcorn (with no added sugar or salt), drained well

½ tsp finely chopped fresh parsley

Large pinch of ground turmeric

1 tbsp full-fat crème fraîche

Freshly ground black pepper

1. Put the potatoes in a saucepan, cover with water and bring to the boil. Reduce the heat, cover the pan and simmer for 5 minutes, then add the carrot and cook for another 8–10 minutes or until the vegetables are tender. Drain and, when cool enough to handle, peel the potatoes if the skin is thick, or leave unpeeled. Put the potatoes and carrots in a bowl and roughly mash or chop.

2. While the vegetables are cooking, poach the salmon in the milk in another pan with the sweetcorn for 8 minutes until the salmon is cooked. Stir in the parsley 1 minute before the end.

3. Tip the salmon mixture into the bowl with the vegetables and add the turmeric. Stir in the crème fraîche and a half grind of black pepper. Using the back of a fork, mash the salmon mixture, adding a splash more milk if needed. Alternatively, finely chop.

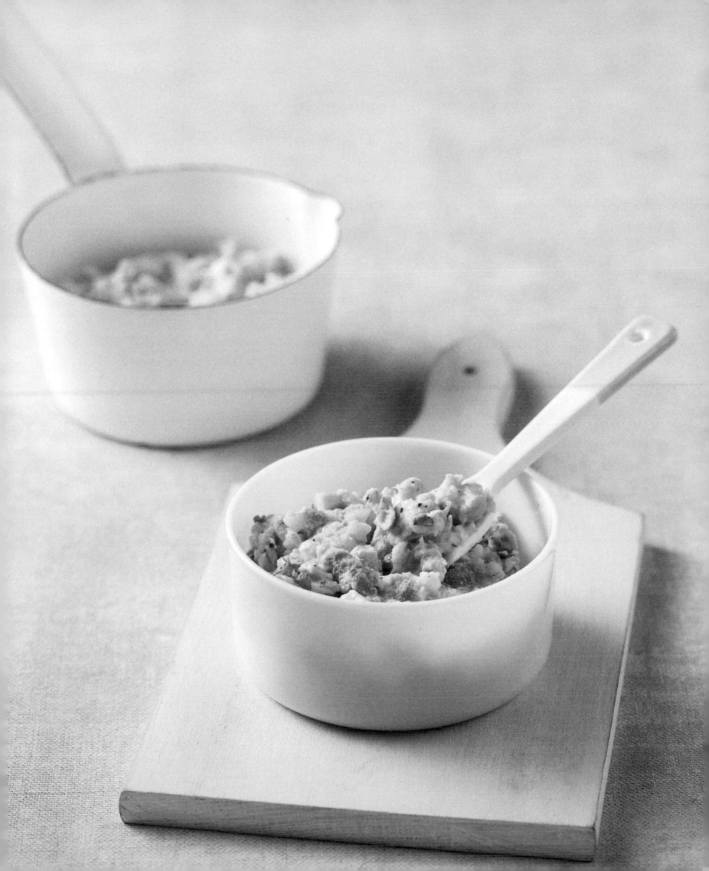

FEEL-GOOD CHICKEN NOODLES

Serves 2–3 (babies/young children) | ❋ *Suitable for freezing*

Healthy chicken soup makes you feel better – fact. This one is packed with immune-boosting kale and ginger, garlic and turmeric, which have been shown to have antibacterial and anti-inflammatory effects.

1 carrot (about 50g/2oz), scrubbed/peeled and roughly chopped

40g/1½oz fine dried egg noodles

1cm/½in piece of fresh root ginger, sliced into rounds as thick as a £1 coin

1 large garlic clove, peeled and cut in half

20g/¾oz kale, tough stalks removed, finely chopped

1 tsp coconut oil

125g/4½oz skinless, boneless chicken breast, cut into small pieces

115ml/4fl oz Chicken Bone Broth (see page 111)

¼ tsp ground turmeric

1. Place the carrot in a food processor or spice/coffee grinder and blitz to a coarse paste.
2. Put the carrot in a saucepan with the noodles, ginger, garlic and kale. Pour over enough just-boiled water from a kettle to cover and then bring back up to the boil. Reduce the heat slightly and cook for 3 minutes or until the noodles are tender, then drain, saving 115ml/4fl oz of the cooking water if not using the broth. Discard the ginger and mash the garlic with the back of a fork.
3. Melt the coconut oil in a small frying pan over a medium heat, add the chicken and fry over a medium-high heat for 5 minutes or until cooked through. Finely chop the chicken and add to the noodle mixture with the turmeric, mashed garlic and broth or saved cooking water. Using the back of a fork, mash the noodle mixture. Alternatively, finely chop.

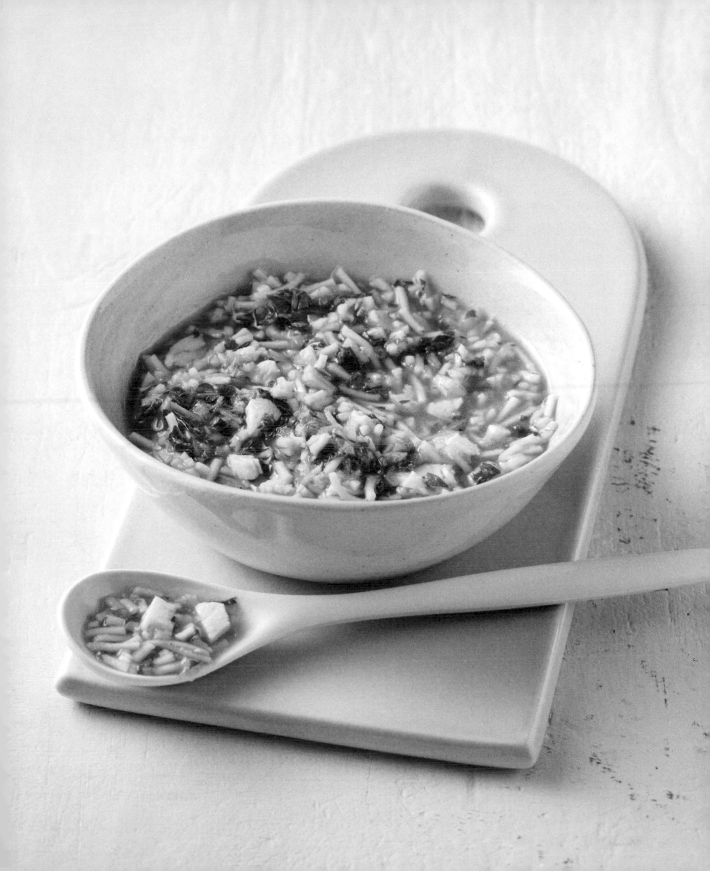

CHICKEN AND SWEET POTATO PARCEL

Serves 2 (baby/young child) | ❋ *Suitable for freezing*

The beauty of this recipe lies in its flexibility, so feel free to add to, or adapt, the content of the chicken parcels depending on your child's likes and dislikes – carrots, fennel, leeks, courgette, peas and seafood all work well. The recipe makes a generous single serving, but do double or triple the amount depending on the number of people you are serving.

75g/3oz sweet potato, peeled and cut into thin rounds

¼ small onion, thinly sliced

1 tbsp chopped red pepper

1 garlic clove, finely chopped

1 tsp olive oil

1 skinless, boneless chicken thigh

3 cherry tomatoes, halved

Large pinch of dried oregano

1. Preheat the oven to 200°C/400°F/Gas 6. Tear off a sheet of foil large enough to make a parcel to hold the vegetables and chicken.
2. Mix together the sweet potato, onion, red pepper, garlic and olive oil in a bowl until combined. Place in the middle of the foil and top with the chicken and tomatoes. Sprinkle over the oregano and add ½ tablespoon of water.
3. Seal the foil parcel, tucking in the edges. Place on a baking tray and bake in the oven for 35–40 minutes. Take a peak in the parcel to make sure the chicken is cooked through – pierce with a skewer to check that the juices are running clear – and the sweet potatoes are tender. If they are not quite done, reseal the parcel and cook for another 5 minutes or so.
4. Open the parcel and transfer everything to a plate, including any juices. Finely chop everything or just chop the chicken and mash the vegetables using the back of a fork.

MILD THAI CHICKEN CURRY

Serves 2–3 (babies/young children) | ❋ *Suitable for freezing*

Aromatic, rather than spicy hot, this is a great introduction to curry. It really pays in the long term to give your baby a wide range of taste experiences, as he is more likely to be accepting of new foods when he's older. Any leftover coconut milk can be used to make the Coconut Fish with Quinoa on page 126.

50g/2oz white long-grain rice, rinsed

1 lemongrass stick (outer layer removed), crushed with the side of a knife

3 tbsp diced red pepper

40g/1½oz small cauliflower florets

2 green beans, thinly sliced

1 tsp coconut oil or sunflower oil

125g/4½oz skinless, boneless chicken breast, cut into small bite-sized pieces

¼ tsp ground turmeric

5 tbsp coconut drinking milk (from a carton), plus extra if needed

1. Put the rice and lemongrass in a saucepan, cover with water and bring to the boil. Turn the heat down to low and simmer, covered, for 5 minutes. Add the red pepper, cauliflower and green beans, and cook for another 5–7 minutes until everything is tender.
2. Meanwhile, heat the coconut or sunflower oil in a frying pan over a medium heat, add the chicken and fry for 5 minutes until cooked through.
3. Drain the rice mixture and return it to the pan, then add the cooked chicken, turmeric and coconut milk, and heat gently to warm through.
4. Using the back of a fork, mash to a coarse purée, adding a splash more coconut milk if needed. Alternatively, finely chop.

PASTA CHEESE WITH NUTTY SPRINKLE

Serves 3–4 (babies/young children) | ❄ *Suitable for freezing*

You can't beat macaroni cheese, but this baby-friendly version is made with orzo (which looks like a cute pasta version of rice) and also includes lots of healthy veg. No lengthy baking is needed as this version is cooked entirely on the hob and comes sprinkled with a nutrient-boosting crunchy nut topping.

100g/3½oz dried orzo pasta

75g/3oz small broccoli florets

1 small leek, finely chopped

15g/½oz unsalted butter

1 tbsp plain flour

200ml/7fl oz full-fat milk, warmed, plus extra if needed

40g/1½oz cauliflower florets, grated

1 tsp Dijon mustard

60g/2½oz mature Cheddar cheese, grated

For the nutty sprinkle

25g/1oz blanched hazelnuts

1 tbsp sunflower seeds

1. Cook the orzo in plenty of unsalted boiling water following the packet instructions, adding the broccoli and leek 5 minutes before the end of the cooking time.

2. Meanwhile, make the nutty sprinkle. Toast the hazelnuts in a large, dry frying pan over a medium-low heat for 3 minutes. Add the sunflower seeds and toast for another 2 minutes, tossing the pan frequently to stop them burning. Place the nuts and seeds in a spice/coffee grinder or food processor and grind until very finely chopped, then set aside.

3. To make the cheese sauce, melt the butter in a saucepan. Add the flour and cook over a low heat, stirring constantly, for 2 minutes. Gradually pour in the warm milk, stirring, then add the cauliflower, increase the heat to medium-low and cook for 5 minutes or until the sauce has thickened to the consistency of double cream. Stir in the mustard and cheese, and cook for another couple of minutes.

4. Drain the pasta and vegetables, and stir them into the cheese sauce.

5. Using the back of a fork, mash the mixture to a coarse purée, adding a splash more milk if needed. Alternatively, finely chop. Scatter over the nutty sprinkle before serving.

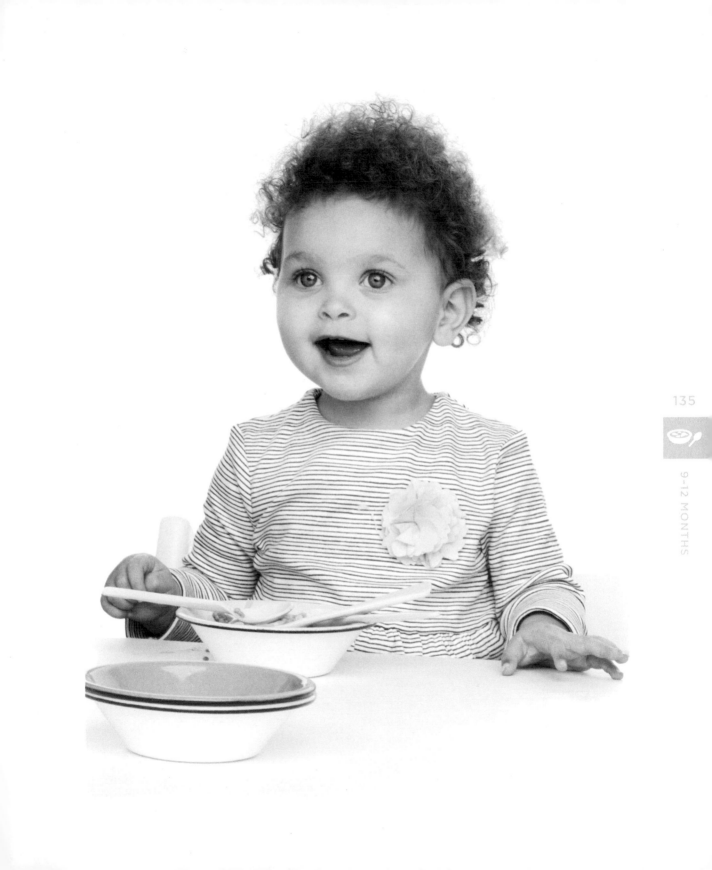

CHINESE PORK AND RICE

Serves 2–3 (babies/young children)

Traditional Chinese flavours add a taste of the exotic to this rice, pork, pineapple and vegetable combo. Pineapple contains the enzyme bromelain, which is thought to aid digestion, while the firm core found running down the centre of the fresh fruit makes a great teething stick – to be on the safe side, never leave your baby alone with finger foods.

40g/1½oz white long-grain rice, rinsed

1 tsp coconut oil

75g/3oz lean pork mince

¼ red pepper, deseeded and finely chopped

25g/1oz white cabbage, finely chopped

½ tsp finely grated fresh root ginger

25g/1oz fresh pineapple (core removed), finely chopped

Large pinch of Chinese five-spice powder (optional)

1. Put the rice in a saucepan and cover with water. Bring to the boil, then turn the heat down to low and simmer, covered, for 10–12 minutes or until cooked. Drain and put the rice in a bowl.
2. While the rice is cooking, melt the coconut oil in a small frying pan, add the mince and red pepper, and cook for 5 minutes, stirring. Add the cabbage, ginger and pineapple and the five-spice powder, if using, and cook for another 5 minutes.
3. Add the mince mixture to the rice, stir in enough just-boiled water from a kettle to make a loose consistency – about 2 tablespoons – then, using the back of a fork, mash to a coarse purée. Alternatively, finely chop.

PORK, POTATO AND APPLE HOTPOT

Serves 3–4 (babies/young children) | ❋ *Suitable for freezing*

The new potatoes in this creamy hotpot are cooked with their skins on. Try to use thin-skinned potatoes, such as Charlotte; you may need to remove the skins otherwise, but it's easier to peel potatoes after cooking.

150g/5oz new potatoes (such as Charlotte; unpeeled), scrubbed and cut into 1cm/½in chunks

1 small apple, peeled, cored and cut into 1cm/½in chunks

1 carrot (about 60g/2½oz), scrubbed/peeled and diced

2 tsp olive oil

100g/3½oz lean pork loin fillets, finely chopped

2 spring onions, finely chopped

1 tsp finely chopped fresh parsley

1 tbsp full-fat crème fraîche

1. Put the potatoes in a saucepan, cover with water and bring to the boil. Reduce the heat, cover the pan and simmer for 5 minutes, then add the apple and carrot, and cook for another 8–10 minutes or until tender. Drain over a bowl, saving 100ml/3½fl oz of the cooking water. When cool enough to handle, peel the potatoes if the skin is thick or leave them unpeeled.
2. Meanwhile, heat the oil in a frying pan over a medium heat, add the pork and spring onions, and stir-fry for 5 minutes or until cooked.
3. Add the drained potatoes, apple and carrot to the pork mixture with the saved cooking water, chopped parsley and crème fraîche, and warm through.
4. Mash to a coarse purée using the back of a fork, or finely chop.

» Pork is a great source of a B vitamin called thiamine, which helps our hearts function properly.

SHOOTING-STAR PASTA WITH LAMB AND AUBERGINE

Serves 2–3 (babies/young children) | ❊ *Suitable for freezing*

Tiny star-shaped pasta is usually used in soups and broths, but it's the perfect size and shape for little ones. Made with lamb, oregano and aubergine, the sauce has a Greek feel to it; you could even stir in some tinned white beans, along with, or instead of, the pasta.

2 tsp olive oil

85g/3¼oz lean lamb mince

½ small onion, diced

5cm/2in piece of aubergine, peeled and cut into small pieces

¼ tsp dried oregano

100ml/3½fl oz passata

100g/3½oz dried star-shaped pasta

1. Heat the oil in a frying pan (with a lid), add the mince, onion and aubergine, and cook over a medium heat for 5 minutes or until the lamb has browned and the vegetables are tender. Add a splash of water, if needed.

2. Add the oregano, passata and 100ml/3½fl oz of water, stir together and when the mixture just starts to bubble, reduce the heat and simmer, covered, for 10 minutes or until the lamb is tender and the vegetables are cooked. Mash the lamb mixture using the back of a fork.

3. While the sauce is cooking, boil the pasta in plenty of unsalted water following the packet instructions, then drain and stir into the lamb mixture. Mash or finely chop again, if necessary.

BEEF AND BARLEY BROTH

Serves 2–3 (babies/young children) | ❄ *Suitable for freezing*

This takes a little while to cook, but demands little attention while it simmers away – just an occasional stir. Perfect comfort food, it's worth making a double batch and freezing it in baby-sized portions for future meals.

2 tsp olive oil

100g/3½oz braising or stewing steak, trimmed of excess fat and cut into small chunks

1 small onion, finely chopped

1 carrot (about 60g/2½oz), scrubbed/peeled and diced

1 parsnip (about 75g/3oz), peeled and diced

½ tsp dried thyme

300ml/11fl oz Beef Bone Broth (see page 110) or low-salt stock or water

40g/1½oz pearl barley, rinsed

100ml/3½fl oz full-fat milk, plus extra if needed

1. Heat the olive oil in a heavy-based saucepan, add the steak and cook over a medium heat for 5 minutes or until the beef is browned all over. Add the onion, carrot, parsnip and thyme, and cook for another 5 minutes, then pour in the broth or stock/water and bring almost to the boil. Turn the heat down to low and simmer, covered, for 50 minutes or until the meat is tender.
2. While, the beef is cooking, put the pearl barley in a separate pan and cover with plenty of water. Bring to the boil, then turn the heat down to low, cover the pan and simmer for 45 minutes or until tender.
3. Drain the barley and add it to the beef mixture, then stir in the milk and warm through.
4. Finely chop or blend briefly to a coarse purée in a food processor or using a hand blender, adding a splash more milk if needed.

SUPERFRUIT SUNDAE

Serves 4 (babies/young children) | ❋ *Suitable for freezing*

A special treat, this triple-tiered fruity pudding has a layer of golden mango and of ruby-red raspberry and is topped with thick Greek yoghurt. It's not difficult to prepare, but it's perfectly okay to make it with just one fruit layer, if that's easier for you.

4 rounded tbsp plain full-fat live Greek yoghurt

For the mango layer

150g/5oz mango flesh, chopped

1 tsp chia seeds

For the raspberry layer

150g/5oz frozen raspberries, partially defrosted

1 tsp vanilla extract

20g/¾oz ground almonds

1. To make the mango layer, purée the mango using a hand blender and tip into a bowl. Stir in the chia seeds and chill in the fridge for at least 30 minutes until the chia seeds swell and the mango thickens.
2. To make the raspberry layer, purée the raspberries using the hand blender and pour them into another bowl (you can press them through a sieve to get rid of the seeds, if you prefer). Stir in the vanilla extract and ground almonds, and chill in the fridge until ready to assemble.
3. To assemble, divide the raspberry mixture among four small, clear plastic beakers or ramekins. Top each with a quarter of the mango mixture and a tablespoon of yoghurt. They can be stored in the fridge for 1–2 days.

CHERRY AND BEETROOT SLUSH

Serves 2–3 (babies/young children) | ❋ *Suitable for freezing*

Teething can be painful and uncomfortable for babies – it's no fun for parents, either – and chilled and frozen foods can bring relief to sore gums. This healthier version of shop-bought iced drinks is a tasty mix of beetroot, apple and cherry.

100g/3½oz frozen pitted dark cherries

100ml/3½fl oz fresh apple juice (not from concentrate)

25g/1oz cooked beetroot (not in vinegar)

1. Take the cherries out of the freezer and let them defrost slightly.
2. Put them in a blender with the apple juice and beetroot, and blend to a slushy consistency.
3. Serve straight away or freeze. If freezing, let the slush soften slightly before serving and scrape with a fork to break it into ice crystals.

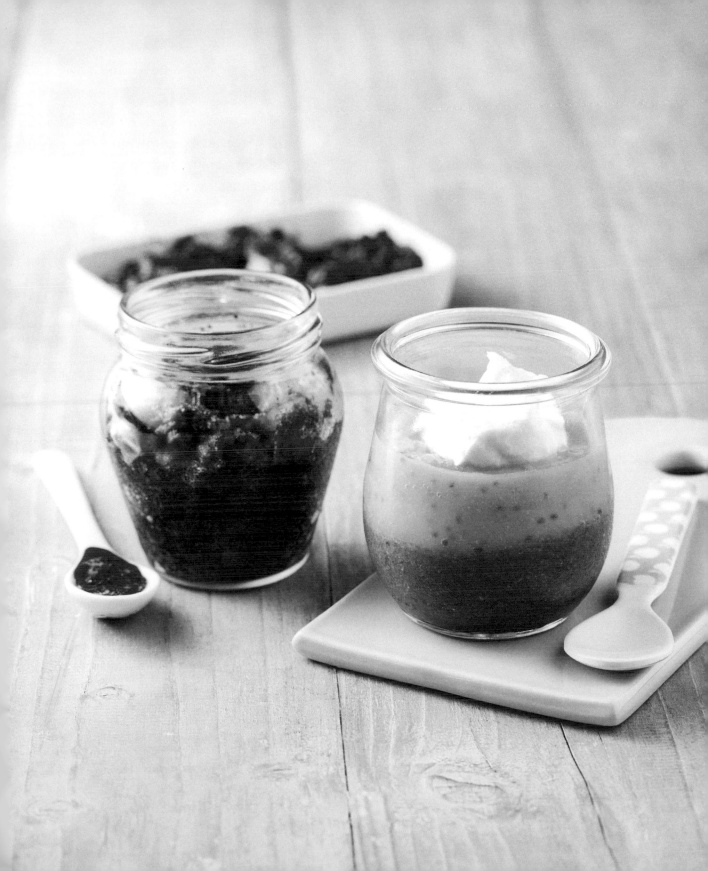

SWEET COUSCOUS PUD

Serves 2–3 (babies/young children) | ❄ *Suitable for freezing*

Couscous doesn't have to be saved for savoury dishes; it makes a comforting alternative to rice pudding when simmered with milk, cinnamon and dates. If you don't have dates, mash a banana into the cooked couscous before serving.

75g/3oz couscous

400ml/14fl oz full-fat milk

3 soft pitted dates, finely chopped

½ tsp ground cinnamon

Put the couscous, milk, dates and cinnamon in a small pan and bring to simmering point, stirring. Cook, stirring frequently, for 10 minutes or until the couscous is very tender. Mash with the back of a fork to crush the grains slightly.

BAKED SPICED APPLE AND SQUASH

Serves 3–4 (babies/young children) | ❄ *Suitable for freezing*

Roasting the squash and apple gives them a lovely sweet caramel flavour, so you don't need to add any sugar.

1 rounded tsp coconut oil or unsalted butter

225g/8oz butternut squash, peeled, deseeded and cut into 1cm/½in chunks

1 large eating apple, peeled, cored and cut into 1cm/½in cubes

½ tsp ground cinnamon

100g/3½oz plain full-fat live yoghurt

2 tsp ground almonds

1. Preheat the oven to 180°C/350°F/Gas 4.
2. Gently heat the coconut oil or butter in a small pan until melted. Add the squash, apple and cinnamon, and stir in the pan until the squash and apple are coated in the spiced oil/butter.
3. Tip the contents of the pan into a baking tray, spread out evenly and roast in the oven for 30–35 minutes, turning halfway, until softened and starting to brown. Check towards the end of the cooking time and remove any pieces of squash or apple that are ready, so that they don't burn.
4. Put the squash and apple in a food processor, or use a hand blender, with the yoghurt and ground almonds and blend until smooth.

AVOCADO AND KIWI

Serves 1 (baby/young child)

Packed with immune-boosting vitamin C, this creamy, zingy fruit purée takes just minutes to make. Add a spoonful or two of live plain yoghurt, if you like, to calm the flavour of the kiwi if it's too sharp.

Flesh of ½ small ripe avocado

1 ripe kiwi fruit, halved and flesh scooped out

Squeeze of lemon juice

Using the back of a fork, mash the avocado, kiwi and lemon juice together until smooth. Alternatively, blend in a food processor or using a hand blender. Serve straight away or spoon into an airtight container to eat later in the day.

PEACH AND RASPBERRY CREAM

Serves 1–2 (babies/young children)

Ground almonds and yoghurt boost the protein content of this creamy fruit mixture. Protein is crucial for the growth and repair of the body's tissues and for the maintenance of good health.

1 ripe peach

60g/2½oz raspberries

2 tsp ground almonds

2 tbsp plain full-fat live Greek yoghurt

½ tsp ground flaxseeds/linseeds (optional)

1. To remove the skin from the peach, place it in a bowl of just-boiled water and leave for 30 seconds. Using a slotted spoon, remove the peach and rinse it briefly under cold running water. Peel off the skin, then halve the peach and remove the stone.
2. Place the peach in a food processor with the raspberries, ground almonds and yoghurt, or use a hand blender, and blend until smooth, then stir in the flaxseeds (if using).

PINEAPPLE, CUCUMBER AND COTTAGE CHEESE

Serves 1 (baby/young child)

Pineapple and cottage cheese are a bit old-school but you can't beat old favourites. Here, they are joined by cucumber and ground flaxseeds to make a simple, no-cook meal. You can remove the cucumber skin, if you prefer.

40g/1½oz pineapple flesh, chopped

1.5cm/⅝in piece of cucumber, quartered, deseeded and chopped

50g/2oz full-fat cottage cheese

¼ tsp ground flaxseeds/linseeds

Using a hand blender, purée the pineapple and cucumber until almost smooth. Add to the cottage cheese and stir or mash using the back of a fork. Finally, stir in the ground flaxseeds.

TUNA, CUCUMBER AND BEANS

Serves 1 (baby/young child)

This makes use of everyday store-cupboard staples to create a simple, no-cook meal. Blended to a smooth purée, it would also make a nutritious dip or topping for toast fingers, crackers or rice cakes.

25g/1oz tinned tuna steak in olive oil, drained

2.5cm/1in piece of cucumber, quartered, deseeded and chopped (peeled if you like)

25g/1oz tinned white beans, drained and rinsed

Flesh of ½ small ripe avocado

Squeeze of lemon juice

Blitz all the ingredients briefly in a food processor, or using a hand blender, to make a coarse paste.

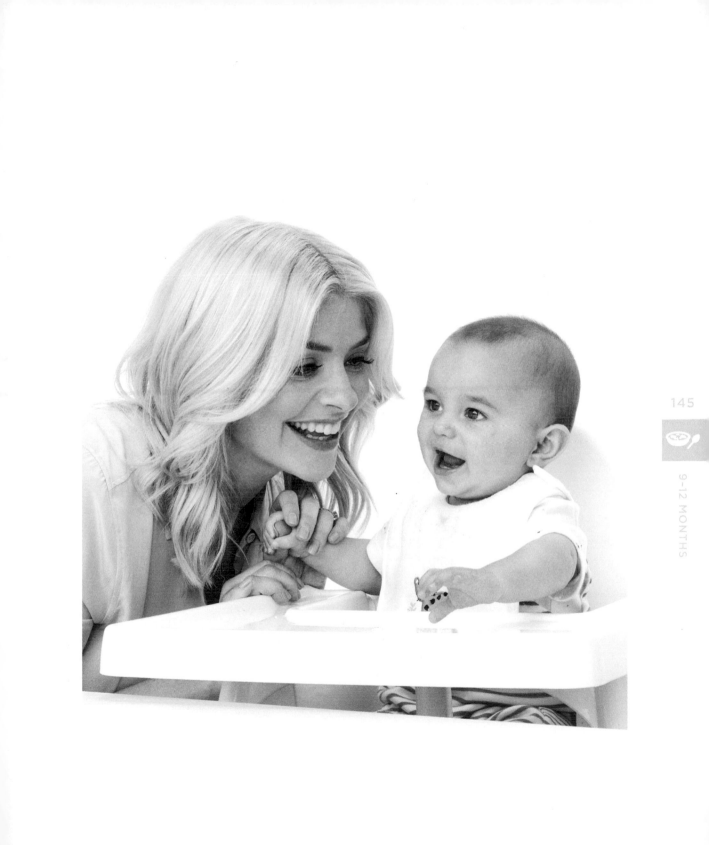

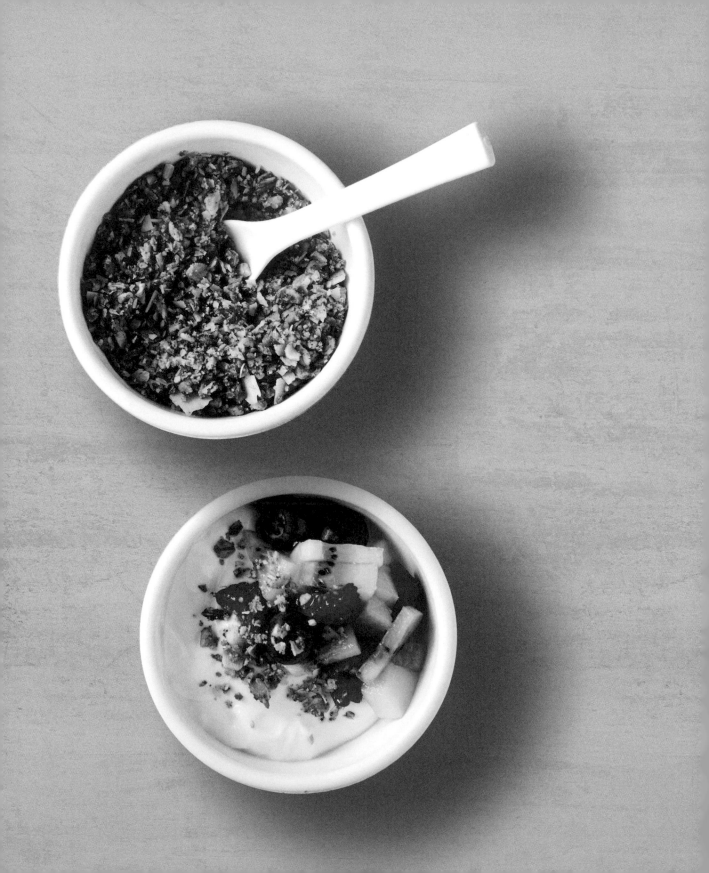

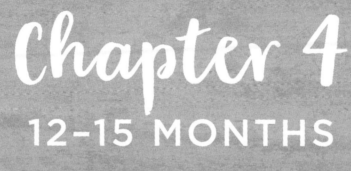

Chapter 4

12–15 MONTHS

In an ideal world, by this stage your baby will be eating pretty much what the rest of the family eat at mealtimes, or some variation of it. As with the previous chapter and Chapters 5–8, I've included lots of recipes that are suitable for the whole family. Veggie Bolognese (see page 169), for example, is a firm favourite in our house, especially on busy weekday evenings. Indian Shepherd's Pie (see page 177) always goes down well, too. With any of these meals, it's crucial to hold off seasoning (especially when it comes to spices!) until after you've removed your baby or toddler's portion.

Sharing the same dish also makes it much easier for everyone to sit together at mealtimes. Your baby is definitely starting to feel like a big girl by this age and will really benefit from sitting down to eat with the rest of the family as often as possible. It's nature's way for babies and children to learn by example, so what better way for them to explore food than sitting beside you at the dinner table. What's that saying? 'Families that eat together, stay together.' I think this is so true. No matter what age your children are – and it might take some years for them to share your appreciation of sitting down together at every meal – dinnertime is family bonding time.

BATCH COOKING

Just because your baby has moved on from purées doesn't mean that batch cooking goes out the window – thank goodness, because it's such a godsend! When you're a busy parent, you don't always have the time to be preparing different dishes all the time and every day of the week.

In this chapter, I've included some of my favourite recipes that also work when prepared in one big batch. They're versatile, too. Breakfasts in my house regularly feature my Gingerbread Granola (see page 152) because it's just so easy to whip up a load of it and store in the cupboard; not just for baby but for the whole family. I often find myself snacking on it in the afternoon, much as I try not to. I try (not always successfully!) to set aside some time at the weekend to prepare big batches of Healthy Alphabet Soup (see page 158) for super-simple lunchtime meals during the week, or Veggie Bolognese (see page 169) for those hectic weekday evenings when the prospect of cooking something from scratch is just too much!

There should be no more puréeing once your baby reaches her one-year milestone. If possible, the food on her plate should resemble your own, just cut up smaller. Some babies seem to be slightly more gluttonous than others. Belle, for example, could manage pretty much a whole plate of something she particularly liked, such as Baked Sweet Potatoes with a topping (see page 166), whereas Harry could barely manage half before getting too full. As long as you're giving your baby nutritious meals and she's a healthy weight, you can be confident that she's getting everything she needs. By the time they reach one year, babies

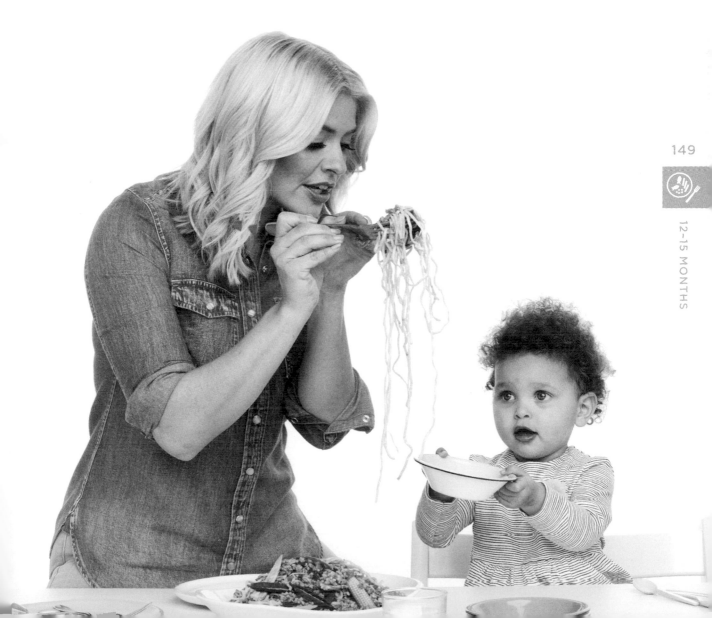

have usually developed a sense of independence. Individual portions of food go down really well – Chicken Pot Pies (see page 174) were popular with all three of mine and really buoyed up their burgeoning sense of individuality!

BREASTFEEDING/MILK

At 12 months, you can move your baby on from formula to pasteurized cow's milk, or continue breastfeeding. If you choose to stop breastfeeding, around 400ml/14fl oz of whole milk a day is recommended. If you switch to cow's milk, make sure it's full fat, however; you shouldn't move your child on to semi-skimmed milk until she is two. And don't offer 1 per cent or skimmed milk until your child is five years old. Little children need the calories and good fat that whole milk provides. It's also got more nutrients than the low-fat versions.

When it came to switching to cow's milk, each of my children reacted differently. Harry wasn't that keen at first, as the flavour is so different, less sweet than formula, so I started mixing formula with cow's milk, 50:50 to begin with and then gradually decreasing the amount so that eventually he was just having pure cow's milk and enjoying it. Belle flat-out refused cow's milk and no matter what tricks I used, she just wasn't interested, so I just upped all the other dairy products she did like to ensure she was still getting enough calcium, being mindful not to feed her too much cheese as it's particularly high in saturated fat! I think by the time your baby is a year old, so long as she's eating a well-balanced diet, you don't need to keep pushing something she's just not keen on.

By contrast, Chester switched to cow's milk from day one without any complaint at all, which might seem bizarre on the face of it given that he had such a bad relationship with milk feeds due to his severe reflux (see page 38). During his first year, I tried everything from breast milk to half a dozen other recommended special 'reflux' formulas, so maybe his taste buds were used to adapting to different flavours. That might also explain why he eats literally anything now, which has been super-helpful for weaning more generally.

The name of the game, as ever, is flexibility. Allow yourself to be guided by the unique wants and needs of your own baby. At one year, you might also want to think about taking away her bottle. It can be difficult, but if you start by giving her cow's milk from a sippy cup (see page 28) instead of her usual bottle, she should associate the change in flavour with the new experience of the sippy cup and accept it more readily. Bottle teats can be detrimental to emerging teeth, so it's important to move on as soon as possible.

SAMPLE MENU

🕐	**Breakfast**	Plain full-fat live yoghurt sprinkled with some Gingerbread Granola (see page 152) and half a chopped-up banana
🕐	**Mid-morning**	Baby's usual milk feed, and Seedy Breadsticks with Roasted Carrot Hummus (see pages 198 and 197) as a snack
🕐	**Lunch**	Baked Sweet Potatoes with a topping of your choice (see page 166), with some cooked broccoli florets or red pepper sticks on the side
🕐	**Mid-afternoon**	Chopped fresh fruit and a rice cake
🕐	**Teatime**	Try a family meal of Sunshine Dhal, with a spicy topping for the adults (see page 165), followed by a Fruity Yoghurt Finger (see page 205) or Peach and Raspberry Cream (see page 143)
🕐	**Bedtime**	Baby's usual milk feed

GINGERBREAD GRANOLA

Makes 275g/10oz granola

Aromatic spices such as cinnamon and ginger have a natural sweetness, which helps to reduce the sugar content of this homemade granola, making it much lower than many shop-bought alternatives. Feel free to swap my choice of nuts, seeds and grains with your family's favourite combination; just keep the ratios similar. Serve stirred into yoghurt or milk with fresh or dried fruit mixed in.

50ml/2fl oz coconut oil

2 tbsp maple syrup

100g/3½oz jumbo porridge oats

75g/3oz pecan nuts, roughly broken

50g/2oz sunflower seeds

2 tsp ground cinnamon

1 tsp ground ginger

40g/1½oz coconut flakes

1. Preheat the oven to 170°C/325°F/Gas 3 and line a baking tray with baking paper.
2. Melt the coconut oil in a small pan over a low heat, then remove from the heat and combine with the maple syrup. Mix together the oats, pecans, sunflower seeds, cinnamon and ginger in a large bowl. Pour the oil and syrup mixture into the bowl and stir until everything is mixed together.
3. Spread the oat mixture out on the lined baking tray and toast in the oven for 20 minutes. Remove the tray, stir in the coconut flakes and return to the oven for another 4 minutes or until the coconut is starting to turn golden. Remove the granola from the oven and leave to cool and crisp up.
4. Depending on the age of your baby and how many teeth she has, it may be a good idea to grind the granola in a food processor to make it easier to eat and reduce the risk of choking.

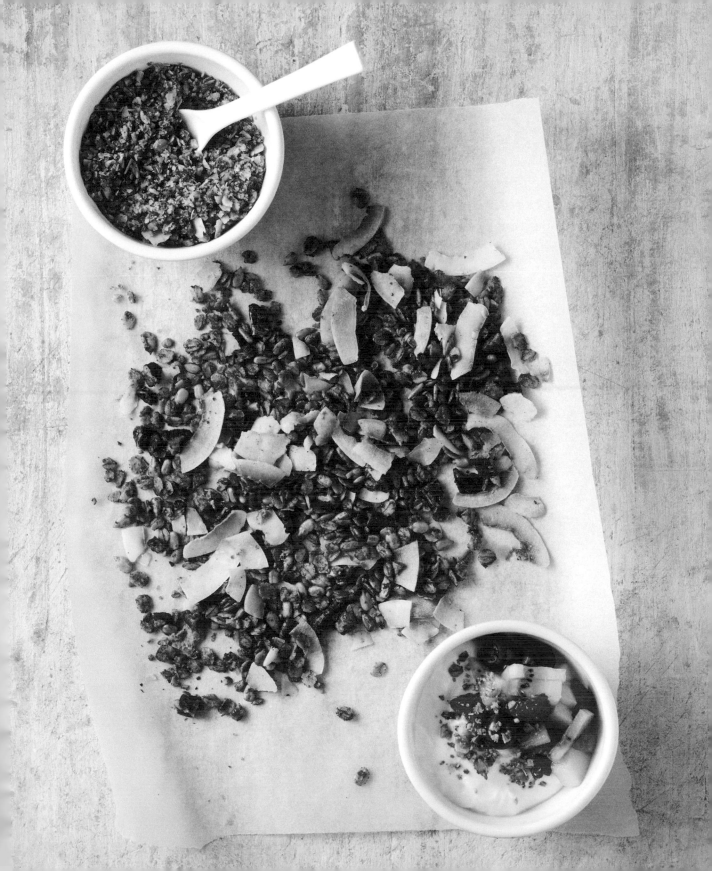

GOOD MORNING PANCAKES

Makes about 8 pancakes | ❄ *Suitable for freezing (pancakes only)*

Great for a weekend brunch (or lunch), these pancakes-cum-fritters make a satisfying start to the day and, thanks to the high protein content of the peas, keep everyone full for the morning ahead. They are topped with a poached egg, but smoked salmon and a spoonful of soured cream is also a winner. Just remember that smoked salmon is salty, so only give little ones a very small amount.

15g/½oz unsalted butter

100ml/3½fl oz full-fat milk

1 large egg

100g/3⅓oz self-raising flour

1 large spring onion, finely chopped

100g/3½oz frozen (and defrosted) petits pois

25g/1oz mature Cheddar cheese, grated

Sunflower oil, for cooking

To serve

4 eggs and/or 75g/3oz smoked salmon slices

3 tbsp full-fat soured cream

1. Melt the butter in a saucepan over a low heat, then transfer to a blender. Add the milk, egg, flour, spring onion and half the peas, and blend well to make a thick, smooth batter. Leave to rest for 15 minutes. Just before cooking, stir in the cheese and the remaining peas.

2. Pour in enough of the sunflower oil to coat the base of a large frying pan and place over a medium heat. Add 3 tablespoons of the batter per pancake to the pan, to make four pancakes in total. Cook for 2 minutes on each side or until set and golden, then place on kitchen paper and keep warm on a plate in a low oven while you cook the second batch. The batter makes about eight pancakes in total.

3. To poach the eggs (if using), pour enough just-boiled water from a kettle into a large shallow pan so that it is three-quarters full. Heat almost to boiling, then reduce to a gentle simmer and swirl the water in a clockwise direction. Crack one of the eggs into a small bowl and slip it carefully into the pan, then repeat with the other eggs. Poach for about 3 minutes or until the white of each egg is set and the yolk remains slightly runny – you may wish to cook your baby's egg slightly longer so the yolk is firm.

CONTINUES ON NEXT PAGE

4. Divide the pancakes among four plates and add the smoked salmon slices (if using). Using a slotted spoon, remove the eggs from the pan, allow to drain for a moment on kitchen paper, then place one on top of each portion of pancakes. Serve each plate with a dollop of the soured cream.

CARROT 'CAKE' OATS

Serves 2 (young children)

The flavour of this twist on Bircher muesli, or overnight oats, reminds me of carrot cake! Soaking the oats first – and you can also do this before making porridge – is believed to make them easier to digest and their nutrients more readily absorbed.

40g/1½oz rolled porridge oats

200ml/7fl oz full-fat milk (unsweetened almond or cow's milk), plus extra if needed

1 tbsp ground almonds

1 small carrot (about 25g/1oz), scrubbed/peeled and finely grated

1 small eating apple, peeled, cored and grated

¼ tsp ground mixed spice

A few blueberries

1 tbsp very finely chopped nuts and seeds (optional)

1. Put the oats in a bowl, pour over the milk and stir in the ground almonds until combined. Cover and leave in the fridge overnight.
2. The next day, stir in the carrot, apple and mixed spice, and serve with a few blueberries scattered over the top and a splash more milk, if you think it's needed. You could top the oat mixture with a scattering of very finely chopped nuts and seeds, if you like.

BAKED AVOCADO NESTS

Serves 2 (young children)

With their creamy, mashable texture, avocados are perfect for little ones. If you're serving for adults, you could spice this up with a sprinkling of finely chopped red chilli.

1 ripe avocado, halved and stone removed

2 small eggs

1 tomato, deseeded and diced

Squeeze of lemon juice

Olive oil, for drizzling

2 slices of wholemeal bread, toasted, to serve

1. Preheat the oven to 180°C/350°F/Gas 4.
2. Using a teaspoon, scoop out (and eat!) some of the middle of the avocado to make room for the egg. Place the avocado halves in a small baking tray and scrunch up some foil around them to keep them upright and stable.
3. Crack an egg into a jug and tip it into the hollowed-out space in one of the avocado halves. Scatter over half of the diced tomato, then add a little lemon juice and a drizzle of olive oil. Repeat with the second avocado half and egg.
4. Bake the avocado halves in the oven for 20–25 minutes or until the eggs are cooked. Serve with the toast and a spoon for eating the egg and avocado. Alternatively, scoop out the filling and mash with the back of a fork, spreading it on top of the toast, if you like.

» Avocados are packed full of good fats, vitamins and minerals and eggs are a great source of protein, making this a perfect nutrient-laden breakfast-cum-brunch for your little one.

BREAKFAST HASH

Serves 4 (2 young children + 2 adults)

This is perfect for using up leftover cooked potatoes and veg, especially from a roast dinner. And feel free to swap the cabbage and sprouts with whatever's lurking in the fridge – cooked broccoli, peas, beans, cauli or carrots are all good – provided they haven't been seasoned. For the grown-ups, a squirt of sriracha chilli sauce doesn't go amiss.

1 tbsp olive oil

450g/1lb cooked potatoes, cut into 1.5cm/⅝in chunks

75g/3oz lightly cooked green cabbage, shredded

50g/2oz lightly cooked Brussels sprouts, thinly sliced

3 tomatoes, deseeded and diced

½ tsp mild smoked paprika

4 eggs

1. Heat the oil in a large frying pan over a medium heat, add the potatoes and cook for 7 minutes or until starting to turn golden. Stir in the cabbage, Brussels sprouts and tomatoes, adding a splash of water if the mixture seems too dry, and cook for another 5 minutes, turning the vegetables frequently and squashing them down with the back of a spatula. Stir in the smoked paprika – or save this for the adult portion of the dish, if you prefer.

2. Meanwhile, poach the eggs. Pour enough just-boiled water from a kettle into a large shallow pan so that it is three-quarters full. Heat almost to boiling, then reduce to a gentle simmer and swirl the water in a clockwise direction. Crack one of the eggs into a small bowl and slip it into the pan, then repeat with the other eggs. Poach for about 3 minutes or until the white of each egg is set and the yolk remains slightly runny – you may wish to cook your baby's egg slightly longer so the yolk is firm.

3. Divide the hash among four plates. Using a slotted spoon, remove the eggs from the pan, allow to drain for a moment on kitchen paper, then place an egg on top of each serving of hash. Finely chop or mash your baby's portion.

HEALTHY ALPHABET SOUP

Serves 4 (2 young children + 2 adults)

This reminds me of a well-known tinned tomato soup, though my version is loaded with extra veggies and cannellini beans, which help to thicken the soup as well as adding more nutrients.

2 tbsp olive oil

1 large onion, finely chopped

1 large garlic clove, finely chopped

1 celery stick, finely chopped

2 carrots, scrubbed/peeled and coarsely grated

400g/14oz tin of cannellini beans, drained and rinsed

500ml/18fl oz passata

500ml/18fl oz low-salt vegetable stock (for homemade Vegetable Stock, see page 109)

1 tsp dried oregano

100g/3½oz alphabet-shaped dried pasta

2 tbsp full-fat crème fraîche

1. Heat half the oil in a large saucepan, add the onion, garlic, celery and carrots, and cook for 5 minutes until softened.
2. Tip in the beans and stir in the passata, stock and oregano. Heat until the soup starts to bubble, then turn the heat down, partially cover the pan and simmer for 20 minutes, stirring occasionally.
3. Just before the soup is ready, boil the pasta until al dente in plenty of unsalted water following the packet instructions. Remove from the heat, drain and toss in the remaining olive oil to stop the shapes sticking together.
4. Using a hand blender, blend the soup until smooth, then stir in the crème fraîche. Ladle the soup into four shallow bowls and serve with the pasta scattered over the top or stirred in.

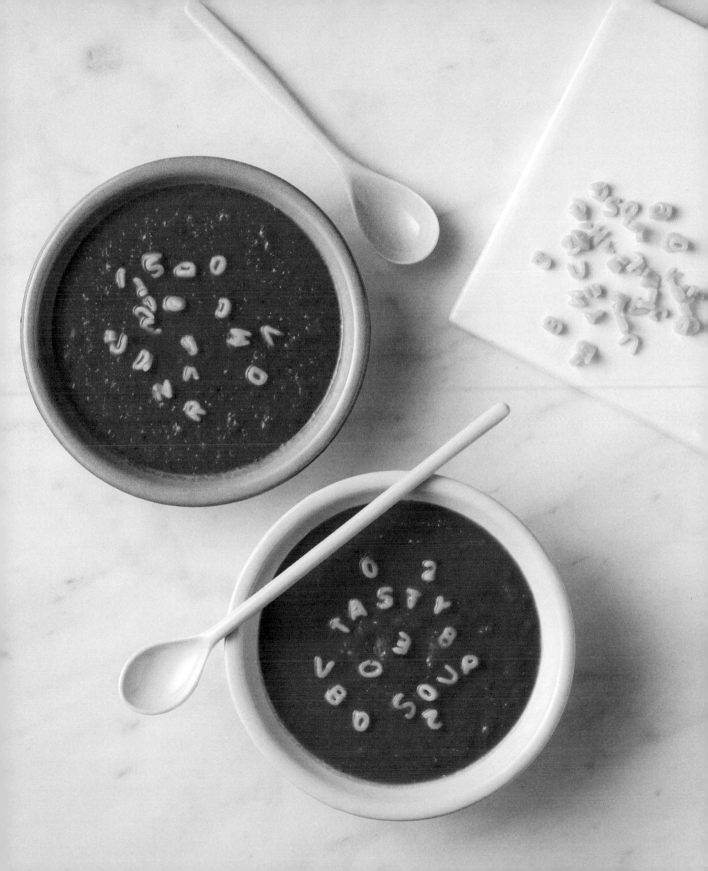

TASTY THINGS ON TOAST

Each serves 2 (young children)

Quick and nutritious, these simple topping ideas take toast to a new level.

EDAMAME BEANS ON GARLIC TOAST

This pretty pale-green edamame and ricotta spread is delicious on garlicky toast. You can find edamame (or soya) beans in the freezer section of large supermarkets or Asian grocers.

75g/3oz frozen edamame beans

50g/2oz ricotta cheese

1 spring onion, chopped

1 large handful of fresh mint leaves

Juice of ½ unwaxed lemon and ½ tsp finely grated zest

Splash of full-fat milk (optional)

For the garlic toast

2 slices of crusty wholegrain bread

1 small garlic clove, peeled and cut in half

Extra-virgin olive oil

1. Place the edamame beans in a saucepan and cover with water. Bring to the boil, then reduce the heat, cover the pan and boil for 5 minutes or until tender. Drain the beans and cool under cold running water.
2. Put the beans in a blender or food processor with the ricotta, spring onion, mint, lemon juice and zest, and blend until smooth and creamy. Add a splash of milk if the mixture is too thick – you want it to be a thick but spreadable consistency.
3. Toast the bread in a griddle pan over a medium-high heat (or use a toaster) and toast on each side until crisp and golden. Rub each slice with the cut side of the garlic and drizzle over a little olive oil. Cut the toast into quarters and top with a layer of the bean mixture.

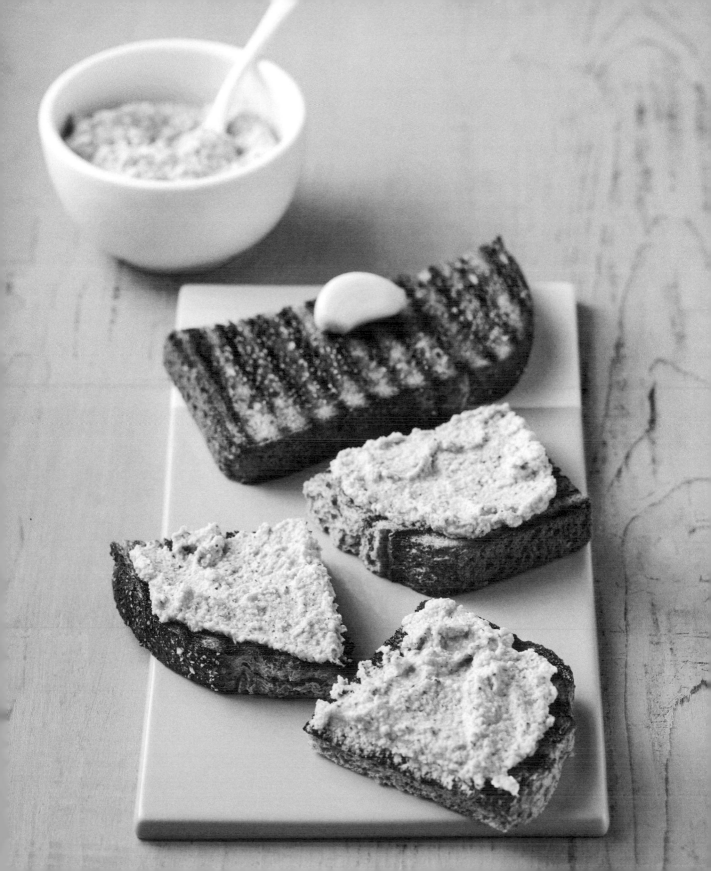

CAULI CHEESE ON TOAST

Children can find cauliflower bitter, but combine the vegetable with dairy foods and it's a different story. In fact, in this twist on the ever-popular cheese on toast, it's barely detectable.

2 slices of wholemeal bread

1 large egg yolk

4 tsp full-fat milk

40g/1½oz mature Cheddar cheese, grated

2 cauliflower florets (about 40g/1½oz in total), grated

Unsalted butter, for spreading

1. Preheat the grill to medium-high and lightly toast one side of each slice of bread.
2. Meanwhile, beat together the egg yolk and milk in a bowl and stir in the cheese and grated cauliflower, crushing the cauliflower slightly with the back of a fork.
3. Butter the untoasted side of each slice of toast, then spoon the cauli mixture on top, spreading it out to the edge. Grill for 5 minutes or until the cheese mixture starts to turn golden in places. Leave to cool slightly before cutting into squares or fingers.

FISH TOAST FINGERS

Not the usual fish fingers in a breadcrumb coating – these toast fingers are topped with a heart-friendly, omega-3-rich blend of trout and avocado. Find cooked trout fillets (they are normally pink) in the fish section in supermarkets or at a fishmonger's.

2 slices of seedy wholegrain bread

50g/2oz skinless, boneless cooked trout fillet, flaked

Flesh of ½ ripe avocado

2 tsp red pesto

Squeeze of lemon juice

1. Toast the bread under the grill or in a toaster.
2. Meanwhile, put the trout, avocado and pesto in a bowl. Add a squeeze of lemon juice and use the back of a fork to mash to a coarse purée. Spread the trout mixture over the toast and cut into fingers.

CASHEW CREAM AND STRAWBERRY TOAST

Simply yum! Instead of serving the cashew and strawberry cream in pots, as on page 118, it's spread on toasted wholegrain bread. Or you could try brioche as a special treat.

2 slices of wholegrain bread (or brioche as a treat)

½ quantity of the Swirly Strawberry Cashew mixture (see page 118)

3 strawberries, hulled and sliced

Lightly toast the bread under the grill or in a toaster. Spread a thick layer of the strawberry-cashew cream on top and then cut in half or quarters. Top with the sliced strawberries.

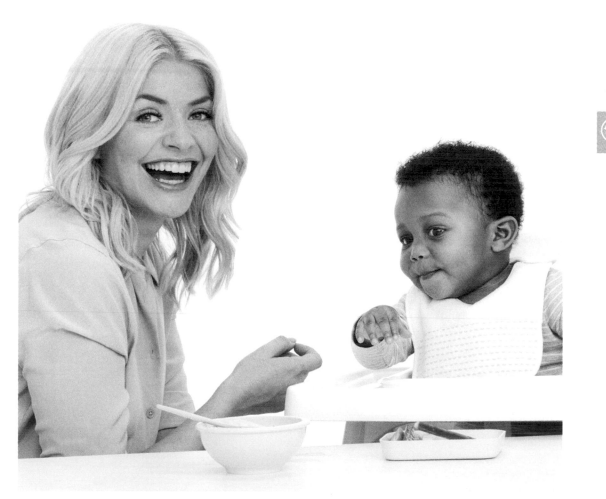

BROCCOLI AND QUINOA BITES

Makes 8 'bites'

Equally delicious served cold or hot, these protein-rich 'bites' make a healthy snack or lunch served with vegetable sticks and a dip. Store, covered, in the fridge for up to three days – if they last that long!

25g/1oz quinoa (100g/3½oz cooked weight)

150g/5oz broccoli florets

1 large spring onion, finely chopped

50g/2oz mature Cheddar cheese, grated

1 egg, lightly beaten

1. First cook the quinoa. Put it in a saucepan, cover with water and bring to the boil. Reduce the heat to low, partially cover the pan and simmer for 15 minutes or until tender. Drain and leave to cool.
2. Preheat the oven to 200°C/400°F/Gas 6 and line a baking sheet with baking paper.
3. Blitz the broccoli in a food processor until very finely chopped and then scrape it into a large bowl. Stir in the cooked and cooled quinoa, the spring onion, cheese and egg, and stir well until combined.
4. Using damp hands, form the broccoli mixture into eight sausage-shaped patties, about 5cm/2in long (the mixture is fairly wet but will hold together when pressed). Place the 'bites' on the prepared baking sheet and cook in the oven for 25 minutes or until firmed up and golden in places.

SUNSHINE DHAL

Serves 4–5 (2–3 young children + 2 adults) | ❋ *Suitable for freezing (dhal only)*

It can be tricky to get kids to enjoy lentils, but the split red variety can be blended until smooth, so no off-putting lumps. This dhal is mildly spiced but comes with a lively topping that perks things up for the grown-ups.

1 large red onion, roughly chopped

1 large carrot, scrubbed/peeled and roughly chopped

2 large garlic cloves, peeled

2.5cm/1in piece of fresh root ginger, roughly chopped (no need to peel)

1 tbsp coconut oil

175g/6oz split red lentils, rinsed

1 tsp ground coriander

1 tsp ground cumin

1 tsp ground turmeric

400g/14oz tin of full-fat coconut milk

400ml/14fl oz low-salt vegetable stock (for homemade stock, see page 109)

2 tomatoes, deseeded and diced

Wholemeal chapattis, to serve

Spicy topping (for the grown-ups – optional)

2 tsp coconut oil

1 tbsp grated fresh root ginger

2 handfuls of kale, tough stalks discarded and leaves finely chopped

1 fresh red chilli, deseeded and diced

2 garlic cloves, chopped

Juice of ½ lime

1. Put the onion, carrot, garlic and ginger in a food processor and blitz to a coarse purée.
2. Melt the coconut oil over a medium heat, add the onion mixture and cook for 5 minutes, stirring. Stir in the lentils, followed by the ground spices, coconut milk and vegetable stock. Heat until almost bubbling, then turn the heat down to low and simmer, partially covered with a lid, for 15 minutes.
3. Stir in the tomatoes and cook for another 5–10 minutes or until the lentils are soft and starting to break down.
4. While the dhal is cooking, make the spicy topping (if using). Melt the coconut oil in a small frying pan, add the ginger, kale, chilli and garlic, and stir-fry for 2 minutes or until tender. Add the lime juice and set aside.
5. Serve the dhal with the chapattis by the side. You could mash the children's portion to a coarse purée using the back of a fork, or blitz with a hand blender to get rid of any hard bits. Add a good spoonful of the spicy topping, if you like.

» Lentils are a great source of zinc – a mineral that helps heal wounds and keep our hair, nails and skin healthy.

BAKED SWEET POTATOES WITH BARBECUE BEANS (AND OTHER TOPPINGS)

Serves 3–4 (young children) | ❊ *Suitable for freezing (barbecue beans only)*

There's something heart-warming about the vibrant colour of sweet potatoes. They're also brimming with nutrients, including the antioxidant vitamins A and C, both brilliant for our immune systems. Here, I've given a glammed-up version of baked beans, plus other topping ideas. It's well worth baking a few sweet potatoes at a time as any that are left over can be turned into a quick dip blended with olive oil, lemon juice, garlic and tahini.

2 sweet potatoes, scrubbed

Grated hard cheese, to serve (optional)

For the barbecue beans

15g/½oz unsalted butter

1 small garlic clove, finely chopped

1 small carrot, scrubbed/peeled and finely grated

200g/7oz tinned kidney beans, drained and rinsed

½ tsp low-salt soy sauce

¼ tsp balsamic vinegar

1½ tsp tomato purée

1. Preheat the oven to 200°C/400°F/Gas 6. Bake the sweet potatoes in the oven for 50–60 minutes, depending on their size, until tender.
2. To make the barbecue beans, melt the butter in a small saucepan over a medium-low heat, add the garlic, carrot and beans, and cook for a couple of minutes. Add the soy sauce, balsamic vinegar and tomato purée, along with 2 tablespoons of water. Bring almost to the boil, then turn down the heat and simmer, partially covered with a lid, for 8 minutes or until the sauce has reduced and thickened and the beans are tender.
3. When the sweet potatoes are cooked, cut them lengthways down the middle and either serve in their skins or scoop out the insides and mash. Using the back of a fork, roughly mash the beans and spoon on top of the baked potatoes or stir into the mashed potato. Add a sprinkling of grated cheese, if you like.

No-cook toppings

* Mix or blend together 25g/1oz of grated hard cheese, one small grated apple or 5cm/2in piece of cucumber, a good squeeze of lemon juice and 2 tablespoons of plain full-fat live yoghurt.

* Blend together 4 teaspoons of tahini, 4 tablespoons of plain full-fat live yoghurt, 2 tablespoons of tinned chickpeas, a good squeeze of lemon juice and a ¼ tsp mild smoked paprika.

* Blend two drained sun-dried tomatoes in oil with 2 tablespoons of full-fat cream cheese and ½ teaspoon of ground flaxseeds/linseeds. Add 1 tablespoon of full-fat milk to make a spoonable consistency.

* Blend one small ripe avocado with 2 tablespoons of hummus and a squeeze of lime juice.

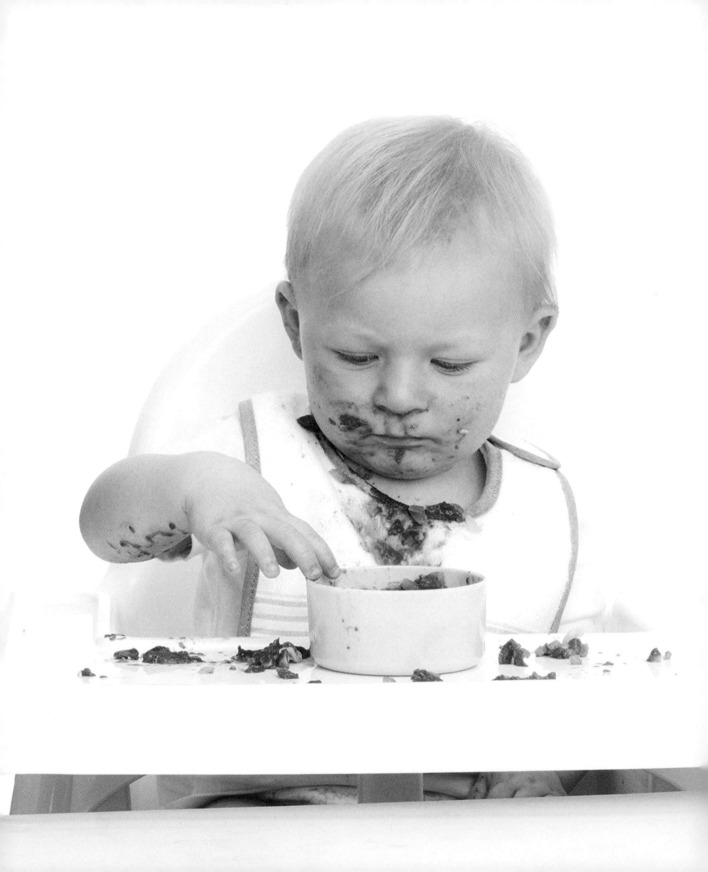

VEGGIE BOLOGNESE

Serves 4 (2 young children + 2 adults)

If your baby isn't keen on mushrooms, try cutting them into small pieces and frying until they start to turn slightly crisp – they become almost bacon-like. As one of the only vegan sources of immune-boosting vitamin D (providing they are grown in sunlight), mushrooms are well worth persevering with.

2 tbsp olive oil

1 large onion, finely chopped

300g/11oz chestnut mushrooms, finely chopped

2 large garlic cloves, finely chopped

400g/14oz tin of chopped tomatoes

150ml/5fl oz low-salt vegetable stock (for homemade stock, see page 109)

3 tbsp basil pesto or Super-veg Green Pesto (see page 124)

280g/10oz dried spaghetti

Freshly grated Parmesan cheese, to serve

1. Heat the oil in a saucepan, add the onion and cook over a medium heat for 5 minutes, stirring often, until softened. Add the mushrooms and cook for another 10 minutes or until they release their liquid and start to turn golden and slightly crisp. Stir in the garlic and cook for another 1 minute.

2. Pour in the tinned tomatoes and stock, and bring to the boil. Stir well, then reduce the heat and simmer, partially covered with a lid, for 10 minutes or until the sauce has reduced and thickened. Stir in the pesto and heat through.

3. Meanwhile, cook the spaghetti in plenty of unsalted boiling water following the packet instructions, then drain over a bowl, reserving 4 tablespoons of the cooking water. Return the pasta to the pan, pour over the sauce and mix until combined, adding some of the reserved cooking water, if needed. Serve sprinkled with Parmesan.

FISH POPCORN AND SWEET POTATO CHIPS

Serves 4 (2 young children + 2 adults)

This healthier version of fish and chips comes with a sugar-free homemade ketchup. The fish pieces are coated in a crisp and golden shell of polenta and sesame seeds, and baked in the oven alongside the sweet potato chips. Peas add the finishing touch.

1 tbsp olive oil, plus extra for greasing

1 tbsp low-salt soy sauce

2 tbsp sesame oil

400g/14oz skinless, boneless thick white fish fillets (such as hake, cod or haddock), flesh cut into 2.5cm/1in cubes

600g/1lb 6oz sweet potatoes, scrubbed, halved and cut into wedges

60g/2½oz sesame seeds

6 tbsp fine polenta

1 large egg

Freshly ground black pepper

For the Quick Tomato Ketchup

100ml/3½fl oz passata

1 tbsp tomato purée

1 tsp olive oil

1 tsp apple cider vinegar

½ tsp Worcestershire sauce

1. Preheat the oven to 200°C/400°F/Gas 6 and grease a baking tray with olive oil.
2. Mix together the soy sauce and sesame oil in a shallow bowl, add the fish and turn until coated. Cover the bowl with cling film and leave the fish to marinate in the fridge until needed.
3. Toss the sweet potatoes in the olive oil and bake in the oven for 35–40 minutes, turning once, until tender and golden.
4. To make the ketchup, put all the ingredients in a small saucepan and cook over a medium-low heat for 5 minutes or until reduced and thickened, then set aside until needed.
5. About twenty minutes before the sweet potato wedges are ready, mix together the sesame seeds and polenta in a shallow bowl and season with black pepper. Beat the egg in a separate bowl.
6. Remove the fish from fridge and discard the marinade. Dip each piece of fish into the beaten egg and then the sesame seed mixture until lightly coated all over. Place on the prepared baking tray and bake in the oven for 10 minutes, turning once, until crisp and golden all over.
7. Serve the fish popcorn with the sweet potato chips and a spoonful of ketchup on the side – don't forget some veg, too!

SALMON FISH BALLS WITH GREEN SAUCE

Serves 4 (2 young children + 2 adults) | ❋ *Suitable for freezing*

Health experts recommend that we eat two portions of fish a week, one of which should be the oily kind, such as salmon, mackerel, sardines, herring or trout. In addition to heart-friendly omega-3 fatty acids, salmon is rich in vitamins B and D. These golden fish balls are a great way of adding oily fish to your little one's diet. Serve with steamed vegetables.

600g/1lb 6oz white potatoes (such as Maris Piper), peeled and quartered

350g/12oz cooked skinless, boneless wild salmon fillets, flesh cut into small pieces

3 tbsp finely chopped fresh parsley

½ leek, very finely chopped

20g/¾oz unsalted butter

1 tbsp Dijon mustard

Plain flour, for dusting

Sunflower oil, for frying

For the green sauce

2½ leeks, finely chopped

250g/9oz frozen peas

125ml/4½fl oz low-salt vegetable stock (for homemade stock, see page 109)

2 tbsp full-fat crème fraîche

1. Place the potatoes in a saucepan and cover with water. Bring to the boil, then reduce the heat, cover the pan and simmer for 15–18 minutes or until just tender (you don't want them to be falling apart), then drain and return to the warm pan to dry. When cool enough to handle, coarsely grate the potatoes into a large bowl. Add the salmon, parsley, leek, butter and mustard, and stir until the butter melts in the warmth of the potatoes.
2. Dust a plate and your hands with flour and form the salmon mixture into 16 balls, each about the size of a large walnut. Set aside while you make the green sauce.
3. Place the leeks and peas in a saucepan, cover with water and bring to the boil. Reduce the heat, cover the pan and simmer for 5 minutes or until just tender – you don't want them to be too soft or mushy. Drain the vegetables and return them to the pan, then add the stock and crème fraîche, and warm through, stirring. Using a hand blender, blend the sauce until smooth and creamy.
4. To cook the fish balls, add enough sunflower oil to coat the base of a large frying pan and place over a medium heat. Add half the fish balls and cook, turning them occasionally, for about 10 minutes until golden and crisp all over. Drain on kitchen paper and keep warm in a low oven while you cook the remaining balls.
5. Reheat the green sauce, if you need to, and serve with the fish balls and some veg.

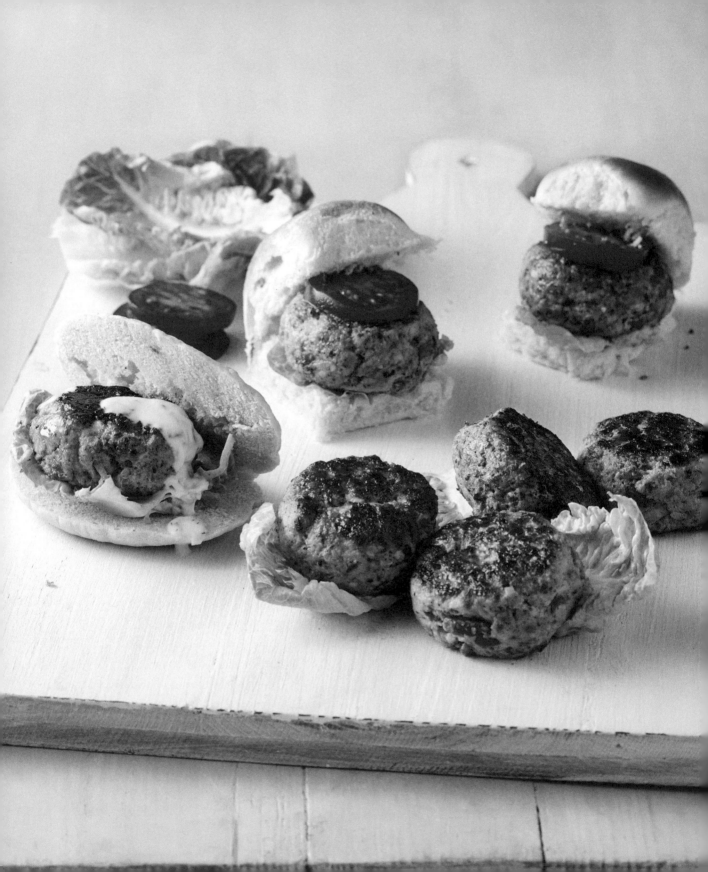

TURKEY AND RED PEPPER BABY BURGERS

Makes 8 burgers | ❋ *Suitable for freezing (uncooked)*

We all love burgers and these mini ones are perfect for babies. They are made with protein-, iron- and vitamin B-rich turkey mince. Here they are served in a bun – or with a bun, for young children – with ketchup, but you could serve them with other favourite accompaniments or as a meal-cum-finger-food with steamed vegetable sticks and pitta bread.

4 seedy oatcakes

1 small onion, chopped

1 large garlic clove, chopped

325g/11½oz turkey mince

75g/3oz roasted red peppers in oil, drained, rinsed and patted dry

½ tsp dried thyme

1 egg, lightly beaten

Pinch of freshly ground black pepper

Sunflower oil, for cooking

To serve

Mini burger buns

Quick Tomato Ketchup (see page 170)

1. Put the oatcakes in a food processor and blitz to fine crumbs, tip into a large bowl and set aside.
2. Put the onion, garlic, mince, red peppers and thyme in the food processor and blend until coarsely chopped. Spoon the mixture into the bowl with the oatcake crumbs and stir in the egg and a little black pepper.
3. With damp hands, form the mixture into eight small burgers; they will be quite wet but will hold together when cooked.
4. Add enough oil to coat the base of a large frying pan and set over a medium heat. Add four of the burgers and fry for 3–4 minutes on each side or until cooked through. Drain on kitchen paper and keep warm in a low oven while you cook the remaining burgers. Serve in/with a bun with ketchup, or finely chop.

» Turkey is packed with nutritional value. It's rich in protein, iron and vitamin B which helps our bodies absorb calcium – promoting bone growth and strength.

CHICKEN POT PIES

Makes 4–6 small pies or 1 large pie | ❋ *Suitable for freezing*

If your baby is troubled with teething – around this age the molars can start to appear – it could be affecting their sleep. Some foods such as chicken (also turkey, bananas, oats and eggs) promote good sleep thanks to the amino acid tryptophan. It may be worth giving these a go . . .

1 carrot, scrubbed/peeled and roughly chopped

2 garlic cloves, peeled

1 celery stick, roughly chopped

1 tbsp olive oil

400g/14oz skinless, boneless chicken thighs, cut into chunks

6 spring onions, finely chopped

75g/3oz button mushrooms, quartered or diced

1 tsp dried thyme

15g/½oz unsalted butter

2 tbsp plain flour, plus extra for dusting

200ml/7fl oz hot low-salt chicken stock (for homemade Bone Broth, see page 111)

60g/2½oz full-fat crème fraîche

375g/13oz ready-rolled puff pastry

1 egg, beaten, or 1–2 tbsp full-fat milk, for glazing

Freshly ground black pepper

You will need 4–6 small ovenproof dishes (about 200ml/7fl oz each) or 1 large dish (about 20 x 30cm/8 x 12in in diameter)

1. Put the carrot, garlic and celery in a food processor and blitz until very finely chopped, then set aside.
2. Heat the oil in a saucepan over a medium heat, add the chicken, spring onions and mushrooms, and cook for 3 minutes. Stir in the carrot mixture and the thyme and cook for another 3 minutes or until the vegetables have softened.
3. Add the butter to the pan and, when melted, stir in the flour. Cook, stirring constantly, for 3 minutes. Gradually pour in the stock, then add the crème fraîche. Season with a little pepper, and cook, stirring occasionally, for 5 minutes or until the sauce has thickened to the consistency of thick double cream.
4. Meanwhile, preheat the oven to 200°C/400°F/Gas 6.
5. Unroll the pastry and cut out rounds large enough to cover the top of the individual dishes, if using, or the single large dish. Re-roll the pastry on a lightly floured work surface, if necessary.
6. Divide the filling among individual dishes or pour into the large dish. Brush the top of each dish with a little egg or milk and lay a pastry round on top, press the edge down to seal and crimp with the back of a fork. Prick the top(s) a couple of times with the fork and brush with more egg or milk, to give the pastry a golden glaze when baked. If using individual dishes, place them on a baking tray. Bake in the oven for 30–40 minutes or until the pastry is cooked and golden.

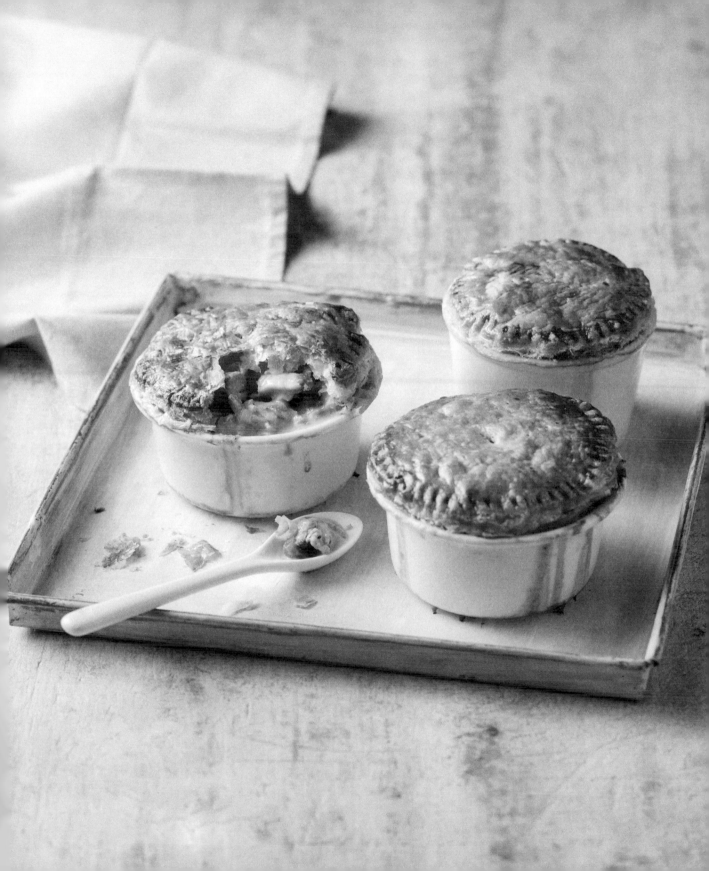

SWEDISH MEATBALLS WITH CRANBERRY JAM AND CREAMY SAUCE

Serves 4 (2 young children + 2 adults) | ❄ *Suitable for freezing (uncooked or cooked)*

Who can resist meatballs, especially served with a tangy cranberry jam and an ever-so-easy creamy sauce. Mash and veg are the perfect sides. It's worth making extra meatballs and freezing them, uncooked, for future meals. They will keep for up to three months.

1 small onion, roughly chopped

1 small carrot, scrubbed/peeled and roughly chopped

50g/2oz rolled porridge oats

350g/12oz lean pork mince

1 tsp wholegrain mustard

½ tsp ground allspice (optional)

1 egg, lightly beaten

Sunflower oil, for frying

For the cranberry jam

100g/3½oz fresh or frozen cranberries

4 tbsp apple juice (not from concentrate)

3–4 (depending on size) soft pitted dates, finely chopped

For the creamy sauce

30g/1¼oz unsalted butter

2 rounded tbsp plain flour

600ml/1 pint hot low-salt chicken stock (for homemade Bone Broth, see page 111)

2 tbsp double cream

1. Put the onion, carrot and oats in a food processor and blitz until finely chopped. Add the pork, mustard, allspice and egg, and process briefly until combined; you don't want to over-process the mince mixture or the meatballs will be tough. With damp hands, form the mixture into balls, each about the size of a walnut – you should have about 22 in total.

2. Add enough sunflower oil to generously coat the base of a large frying pan and cook half the meatballs over a medium heat for 8 minutes or until browned all over. Remove from the pan with a slotted spoon, drain on kitchen paper and set aside while you cook the remaining meatballs.

3. While the meatballs are cooking, prepare the cranberry jam. Put all the ingredients in a small pan and cook for 10 minutes until the cranberries are soft and the mixture has reduced and thickened. Mash the fruit with the back of a fork until almost smooth.

4. To make the creamy sauce, melt the butter in the frying pan (no need to wash it first), stir in the flour and cook over a low heat for 2 minutes, stirring continuously with a wooden spoon. Gradually pour in the stock and cook, stirring, for 5 minutes until thickened, then stir in the cream.

5. Return the meatballs to the pan, spoon over the sauce and heat gently. Serve the meatballs and sauce with a spoonful of cranberry jam on the side.

INDIAN SHEPHERD'S PIE

Serves 4 (2 children + 2 adults) with leftovers | ✳ *Suitable for freezing*

This lightly spiced twist on a family favourite includes lots of veg and is topped with a golden yellow mash – coloured with the wonder spice turmeric. If your little one is sensitive to spices, you can remove a portion of the filling to a small baking dish and make a baby-sized pie. This makes a generous-sized pie – any leftovers can be frozen in portions or will keep in the fridge for up to three days.

1 tbsp olive oil

1 onion, chopped

1cm/½in piece fresh ginger, grated (no need to peel)

325g/11½oz lean lamb mince

1 garlic clove, thinly sliced

1 parsnip, peeled and grated

75g/3oz cauliflower florets, grated

300ml/11fl oz low-salt lamb or chicken stock (for homemade Bone Broth, see page 111)

2 tbsp tomato purée

100g/3½oz frozen peas

2 tsp mild curry powder

1 tsp mild chilli powder (optional)

For the yellow mash

800g/1¾lb white potatoes (such as Maris Piper), peeled and cut into chunks

2 garlic cloves, thinly sliced

1 tsp ground turmeric

60ml/2½fl oz full-fat milk

25g/1oz unsalted butter

1. Heat the oil in a saucepan over a medium heat, add the onion and cook for 5 minutes. Stir in the ginger and mince, and cook for another 5 minutes or until the lamb has browned and the onion is tender.

2. Stir in the garlic, parsnip and cauliflower, then add the stock and tomato purée, and bring to the boil. Reduce the heat, cover the pan and simmer over a medium-low heat for 20 minutes. Stir in the peas.

3. At this stage you can remove your baby's portion, if you prefer, before stirring in the curry powder. Add the chilli powder (if using) to a portion reserved for the adults. Spoon into a large ovenproof dish or separate dishes.

4. Meanwhile, preheat the oven to 200°C/400°F/Gas 6.

5. While the lamb mixture is cooking, place the potatoes and garlic in a saucepan and cover with water. Bring to the boil, then reduce the heat, cover the pan and simmer for 15 minutes or until tender. Drain and return to the warm pan, then add the turmeric, milk and three-quarters of the butter. Warm through and then mash with a potato masher until smooth and creamy.

6. Spoon the mash on top of the mince mixture and spread out evenly. Score the top(s) with the back of a fork and dot over the remaining butter. Bake in the oven for 30 minutes or until the top is golden and crisp. Leave to cool slightly before serving.

PORK WITH PEA GUACAMOLE

Serves 4 (2 young children + 2 adults)

The guacamole sauce not only adds a burst of colour but it's also packed with good things – vitamins, minerals and protein. Here, it is served with a grilled pork loin fillet, but it's equally delicious with lamb or chicken. The sauce also doubles up as a delicious dip, but leave out the added water for a thicker consistency. For an extra kick, grown-ups may like to add an extra crushed clove of garlic to the guacamole.

1 tsp mild smoked paprika

1 tbsp olive oil

4 pork loin fillets

1 large spring onion, thinly sliced on the diagonal, to serve (optional)

For the pea guacamole

225g/8oz frozen peas

2 large garlic cloves, peeled and left whole

Flesh of 1 ripe avocado

Juice of 1 lemon

1. Preheat the grill to medium-high and line the grill pan with foil.
2. Mix together the paprika and olive oil in a shallow dish (you could leave out the smoked paprika for your baby's serving). Add the pork and spoon over the oil mixture until coated.
3. Grill the pork loins for 3–4 minutes on each side, depending on their thickness, until cooked through. Remove from the grill and leave to rest for a couple of minutes or so, covered with foil to keep them warm.
4. While the pork is cooking, make the sauce. Place the peas in a saucepan, cover with water and bring to the boil. Reduce the heat, cover the pan and simmer for 5 minutes or until tender, adding the garlic about 1 minute before the end of the cooking time. Drain over a bowl, reserving 50ml/2fl oz of the cooking water and the cooked garlic.
5. Tip the peas and cooked garlic into a blender, or use a hand blender. Add the avocado, lemon juice and the saved water, then blend to make a smooth and creamy sauce. Either warm the sauce briefly or serve as it is with the grilled pork and with the spring onions sprinkled over, if you like.

RED PEPPER POTS

Serves 4 (2 young children + 2 adults) | ✳ Suitable for freezing (mince filling only)

These roasted whole red peppers have a slight Moroccan feel. The beauty of them is that they can be finely chopped for little ones and served whole for older children and adults. And for those who like a bit of chilli heat, there's a harissa mayo for spooning on top. Serve with a rocket salad.

3 large red peppers

Olive oil, for brushing/greasing

For the mince filling

1 tbsp olive oil

1 large onion, finely chopped

300g/11oz lean beef mince

2 garlic cloves, finely chopped

1 tsp dried thyme

2 tsp ground coriander

1 tsp ground cumin

3 tbsp tomato purée

150g/5oz tinned chickpeas, drained and rinsed

2 tbsp wholewheat couscous

300ml/11fl oz hot low-salt beef stock (for homemade Bone Broth, see page 110)

For the harissa mayo (for the grown-ups – optional)

1 tbsp mayonnaise

3 tbsp plain full-fat live yoghurt

1 heaped tsp harissa paste (or to taste)

Juice of ½ lime

1. Preheat the oven to 200°C/400°F/Gas 6.
2. To prepare the peppers, slice the top third off each one to make a lid and scoop out and discard the seeds. Brush the outside of each pepper and its lid with a little olive oil and place in an oiled baking dish.
3. To make the mince filling, add the olive oil to a large frying pan set over a medium heat. Tip in the onion and cook for 5 minutes until starting to soften, then add the mince and cook until browned, stirring frequently to break it up. Add the garlic, thyme, ground spices, tomato purée and chickpeas, and cook for another couple of minutes. Remove from the heat and stir in the couscous and stock.
4. Spoon the mince mixture into the prepared peppers, putting them close together so they support each other while cooking, and place the pepper 'lids' on top. Cover with foil and bake in the oven for 35 minutes, then remove the foil and cook for another 5–10 minutes or until the peppers are tender.
5. For little ones, cut the pepper in half (half should be enough for a meal) and finely chop. Grown-ups may like to serve the pepper pots with the harissa mayo – simply mix together all the ingredients and spoon on top.

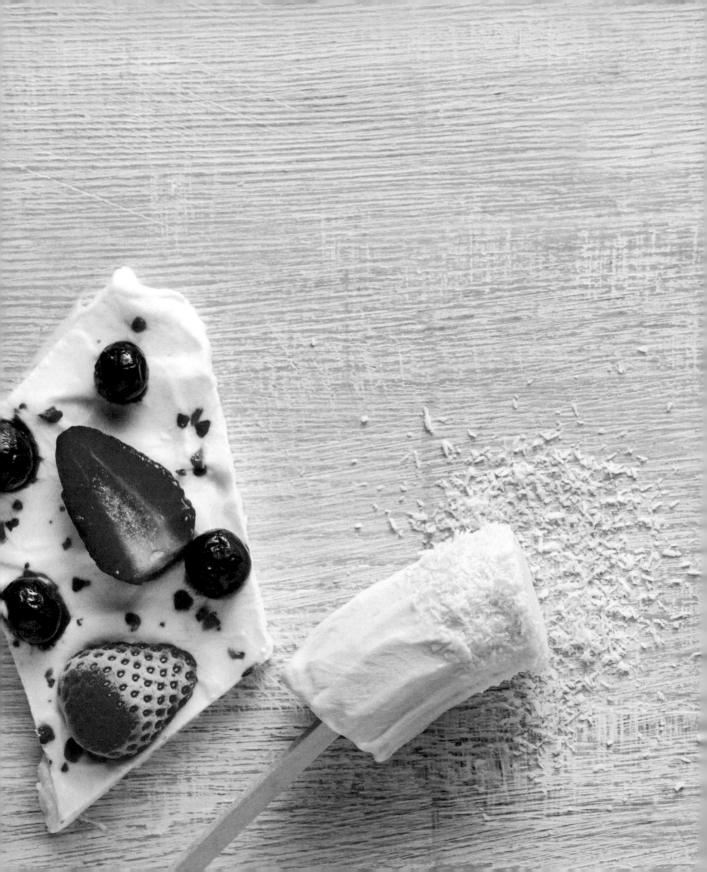

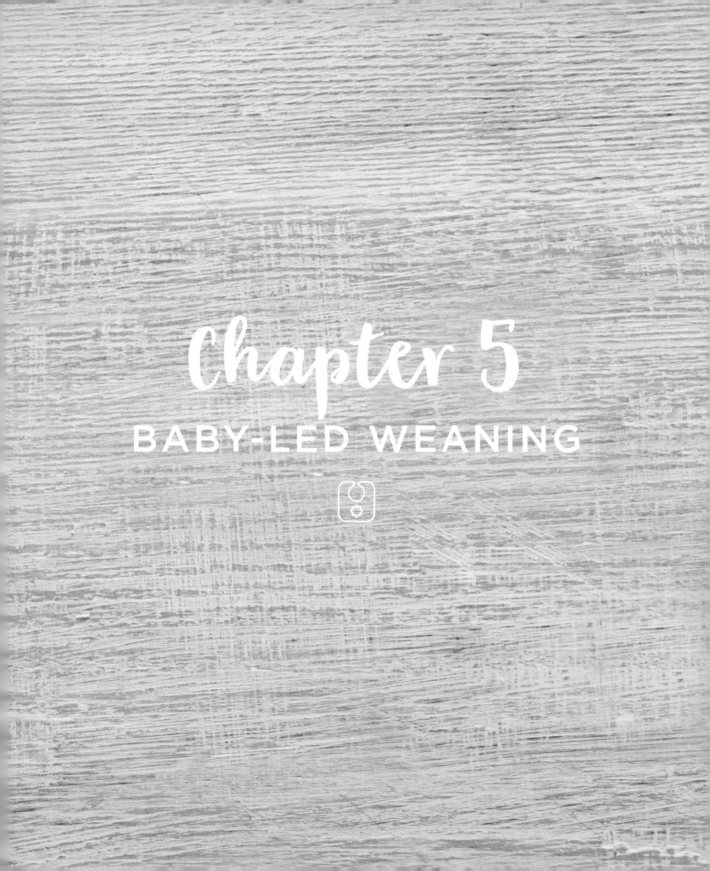

Chapter 5

BABY-LED WEANING

When it comes to weaning, the buzz phrase of the day is baby-led weaning. To spoon-feed or not to spoon-feed! Exclusive baby-led weaning is where babies feed themselves from six months onwards, without any prompting or help from their carer. They are either given finger foods in large stick-shape pieces to be grabbed, squeezed and devoured, or a bowl of food with a small, stubby self-feeding spoon (sometimes pre-loaded), with which they learn to feed themselves, fine-tuning their manual dexterity and hand–eye co-ordination as they go. Babies are free to pick and choose from the range of healthy options with which they are presented, eat at their own pace and stop when they are full. By giving them whole foods presented in pretty much the way nature intended, baby-led weaning is considered an excellent way to educate your baby, quite literally from the start, about fresh, healthy ingredients and what they look and taste like.

Harry and Belle did a bit of both and were as happy to be spoonfed as they were to feed themselves. I did, however, have an exclusive baby-led weaning experience with Chester and it was great. That baby literally led me to baby-led weaning as he refused to be fed purées from a spoon from day dot.

As ever, it's important to note that all babies are different and, as with every new experience, some will take to it like a duck to water and others will be slower to get to grips with it. Equally important is that you continue to give your baby his regular milk feeds to top up whatever he's managing to eat, and that you don't get frustrated and give up. If you commit to baby-led weaning, try to give it every chance. Don't be tempted to start spoon-feeding your baby after a couple of weeks because you're concerned he's not eating enough. He's just adapting to this new way of life. Until now, it's just been, you, him and milk, which you provided without him having to lift a finger. Baby-led weaning takes a little patience for the first few weeks, but persevere – it will be worth it, I promise. It will only be you who's finding it difficult. Your baby will be having a whale of a time getting his hands dirty! In my experience, babies who learn to feed themselves early on develop a healthy interest in food and are less likely to become fussy eaters in later childhood.

Ultimately it is possible to do a bit of both and offer finger foods to spoon-fed children, but unless they've had the opportunity to explore everything for themselves and be fully self-feeding from the start, they may not be as dexterous or have such well-developed mouth muscles or hand–eye co-ordination as a child who's been working hard to feed himself since day one. Spoon-fed babies can be slower to master the art of feeding simply because of being spoon-fed – because you've facilitated the journey from bowl to mouth.

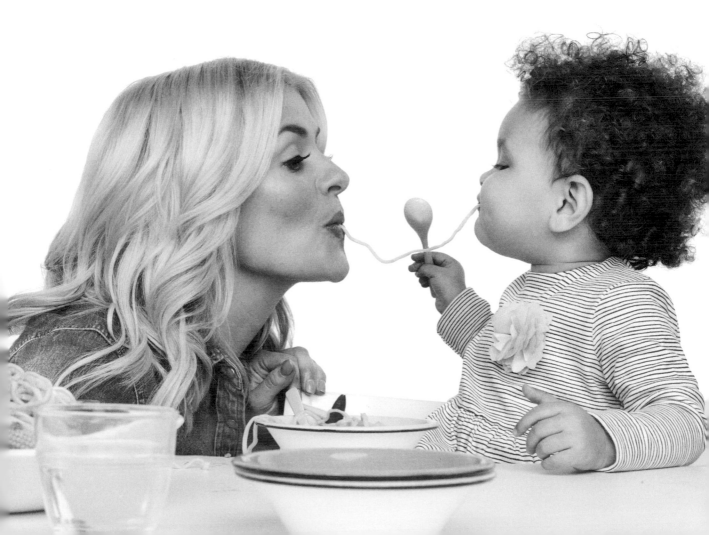

WHY GO BABY LED?

THE PROS

Improved fine-motor skills

Babies who feed themselves are developing their hand–eye co-ordination at every mealtime, meaning that they're getting a lot more practice at it than a spoon-fed baby. Babies will automatically use their hands to begin with, before mastering feeding with a spoon, but that's perfectly normal. It's all part of the weaning experience – and part of the fun!

Greater independence

By letting your little one explore foods for himself, grasping foods in the colours and textures that appeal the most, he will feel more independent. And with every handful he manages to place accurately in his mouth and then swallow, he'll feel a surge of pride and achievement, which can only be good for his self-esteem and confidence.

Eating the same foods as the rest of the family

Not only is this a bonus for the chef, only having to prepare a single meal as opposed to half a dozen 'age-appropriate' ones, but it will also make your baby feel as if he's truly part of the family. This is not only great for building self-confidence but will help him mature more quickly, too, particularly in terms of physical co-ordination. Babies learn by imitation and they will want to copy Mummy and Daddy and any older siblings at the dinner table by trying to feed themselves with their spoon.

Instilling a healthy relationship with food

Baby-led weaning encourages an appreciation for a wide variety of foods and an early understanding about stopping when you are full. Learning self-regulation from such a young age in how much to eat can only be a good thing in a world blighted by weight issues. There's also a lot to be said for raising less fussy eaters this way as they're used to choosing for themselves from a wide range of foods, colours, textures and flavours.

Reduced risk of choking

By letting your baby feed himself, there's less risk of him taking in more than his little mouth can cope with. Babies tend to only pick up as much as they can manage. It's true that, by not puréeing everything and by offering bigger lumps from the start, your baby will most likely spend the first few weeks gagging rather a lot, but he'll learn to chew properly and smash those lumps down to a safe size for swallowing much more quickly than a baby who's spent the first few weeks eating smooth purées. He's simply a more skilled eater, having had far more experience of gumming and sucking food into submission! That said, there still is a risk of choking – see 'Concerns' on page 187.

Good speech training

By feeding themselves from the outset, babies get a lot more practice at learning how to use their tongue to move food around and it's this, combined with the use of all the muscles in their mouth, that's great for their speech development.

Good digestion training

Digestion starts from the moment food is put in front of us. It's the sight, smell and taste of food that gets our stomach juices going, triggering all the enzymes needed to digest it properly when it finally hits the stomach. Touching, tasting and smelling food in the way that baby-led weaning allows – and the fact that the whole eating experience is slowed down while your baby negotiates the complexities of grasping, sucking, chewing and swallowing – makes it the perfect aid to good digestion.

Speedy preparation

With baby-led weaning, you can be more spontaneous about preparing food for your baby as you're knocking out so many steps. Puréeing, mashing, batch cooking, freezing, defrosting, warming and spoon-feeding all take so much longer than boiling or steaming a bit of carrot and broccoli for a few minutes and serving!

Be prepared for the mess!

Babies have a lot to learn when it comes to eating, and experimentation is a messy business. If you're prepared (body bibs, wipe-clean mat, etc.), then it's completely doable. I can't pretend it doesn't make more work for you and sometimes you'll wonder how on earth there's a tomato splat near the top of the door frame, but for me it was worth the grind. You need to think realistically about how patient you are and how much time you have to devote to the process. There's no point in doing it if you're going to get grouchy and frustrated, as babies pick up on atmosphere. If you need to feel more in control, then spoon-feed. And you can always do a bit of both! Every situation, every baby and every carer is different, so choose the method that's right for you and your family.

Fresh foods, cooked from scratch

While you can be more spontaneous about cooking for your baby (see page 185), baby-led weaning involves mainly fresh ingredients, unlike purées, which you can make in batches and freeze. You may need to think ahead more when it comes to shopping for fresh ingredients and to cooking them, especially when your baby is younger and may be eating separately.

A bigger commitment

Everyone involved in caring for your baby has to be on board if you decide that exclusive baby-led weaning is right for you. You can't have anyone spoon-feeding your baby when your back is turned. If your baby realizes there's an easier route from bowl to mouth, it will undo all your hard work! Is your family on board with the level of commitment that will be needed?

Choking risk

Whether you spoon-feed your baby or let him feed himself, there is a prevalent risk of choking, which only lessens as your baby learns the skill of eating safely, that is gumming or sucking food so it's small enough to swallow without gagging or choking. I've read a lot about baby-led weaning, and the general consensus is that there is in fact less risk weaning this way, because children learn to chew more quickly and discover how to intentionally move food to the back of the throat, when it's ready to be swallowed. I don't know how true this is, and I certainly would never take my eyes off a baby when he is eating, no matter what the science says. I think if you're vigilant and have the relevant first-aid knowledge, you're being a responsible parent.

Warning: Always be aware of the choking risk with small whole, round firm foods, such as seedless grapes, blueberries, cherry tomatoes and pitted olives or cherries. Make sure you cut them in half. And peel fruits like apples with tough skins at the beginning, as they are near impossible for toothless mouths to break down.

How much has he actually swallowed?

With so much mess, how can you tell how much your baby has actually eaten? This is not such a concern once you get your head around the fact that, for the first few weeks, eating in this way is a sort of game, to capture his attention and imagination, and generate a love of food. You'll also be continuing with their milk feeds around mealtimes, so he'll catch up with any nutrients and calories he's missing through that. You only start to reduce milk – or be guided by your baby's lack of interest in it – once he starts to consume more than he squishes or drops.

Weight loss

Babies who feed themselves from the word go generally stay at roughly the same weight for the first month or two while they get to grips with eating. But when it does suddenly click – usually towards the end of the eight- or nine-month mark – there's usually a sudden whoosh on the scales as they start consuming loads of goodies. That said, if you are ever concerned about your baby's weight and have noticed a significant drop, consult your GP, or attend your local baby clinic, for a proper diagnosis.

WHEN TO START BABY-LED WEANING

As with spoon-feeding, you can start from roughly six months. Key signs that your baby is ready are that he is sitting up, his tongue-thrust reflex has gone and his gag reflex is under sufficient control that he's able to swallow at least some of the food you're putting in his mouth. You'll find more information about these signs on page 40–1. He should also have a strong fist grasp, which you'll have experienced when you try to prise something he shouldn't have out of that iron grip!

Now, don't expect too much to begin with. You'll find your baby plays with more food than he eats, which is completely normal. He'll still get the bulk of his calories and nutrients from his milk intake during the first few months. Playing with food is all part of your baby literally grabbing this new feeding experience with both hands and exploring food with every sense in his body. By seeing, touching, tasting and smelling foods in more or less their natural state, rather than whizzed up into a purée, his senses will tingle with so much stimulation and it will get his digestive juices going, and if that doesn't spark his interest in solid food, nothing will.

EQUIPMENT

Whether you're spoon-feeding your baby at first or letting him feed himself, you'll need more or less the same basic equipment (see page 43), but there are a few extras that will definitely come in handy.

Self-feeding spoons

Unlike the long-handled spoons you'd buy if you were going down the traditional spoon-feeding route (see page 28), you need to get short fat-handled spoons for your baby to feed himself with. While it's unlikely he'll have the fine-motor skills to be successful with this right away, giving him a spoon to play with while he watches how you use your own cutlery will give him the chance to practise through imitation. Don't be tempted to give your baby a metal spoon. Weaning spoons are made from soft plastic or silicone to be gentle on sensitive gums.

Bowls and plates

Firstly, anything unbreakable. Remember that gorgeous china Peter Rabbit set Grandma bought him for Christmas? Forget it! Put it on display, or store something in it. And, secondly, anything with a suction cup that sticks firmly to the table so your little sucker can't knock it, bang it or throw it without your approval!

Floor mat

Even if your kitchen floor has a wipe-clean surface, you'll probably want to get some kind of wipe-clean, waterproof mat to catch some of the food, which WILL end up on the floor! If you've got wooden floors, getting ground-in food out of the cracks can be a nightmare, and if you've got tiles, you might end up with stained grouting. A lift-up, rinsable mat is far easier to deal with at the end of a messy meal.

There's no need to go out and order an expensive 'weaning' mat, though. In my experience, they're not big enough, anyway, for the surface area that needs covering! Any old plastic sheeting will do. I used a big square of laminated cotton tablecloth for the particularly messy stages – the stuff you can buy by the metre. That way you can get as much or as little as you want. I've even heard of someone using a cheap shower curtain, which I thought was genius. And good old-fashioned newspaper sheets are super-easy as you don't even have to clean them! You can throw the whole lot away and put down another layer for the next meal.

Bibs

There is no contest for what you need here. A bib with sleeves! Preferably one you can run under the tap to clean. If you can't find a bib that doesn't swamp your little one, just go for one that covers as much of his clothes as possible – made from a wipe-clean fabric! I always used those bibs with a tray at the bottom, which is fine if your baby is only having a quick, not-too-messy snack, but absolutely hopeless for a full meal. Still, there's nothing wrong with being an optimist!

As you start weaning around six months, you'll already have got your head around the fact that it's your baby who dictates what and how much they consume, and to a certain extent that applies to their milk feeds too. I say to a certain extent as you'll have to take the lead in the beginning and make sure they are getting enough calories to keep the tummy rumbles away through continuing with their full quota of milk. But as your baby gets better at eating, you'll soon see that he starts to take less milk during the day.

If you're breastfeeding, continue to offer on demand as before, relying on your baby to let you know when he's had enough. You want your baby to be hungry but not starving when you put him in his high chair. And whenever he gives up trying to feed himself because not enough is reaching his tummy, the milk top-up will ensure he won't starve!

After six months and up to 12 months, the recommended daily milk intake for a baby is at least 600ml/1 pint per day. The majority of babies will be desperate for that and some will take more, during the early weaning stages, to supplement what they're not managing to get from food. Until they've learned to chew and swallow solids, milk feeds remain all-important to a baby, but once he starts to master solids, he'll start to take less milk, to the point where he will drop certain feeds altogether.

If your little self-feeder is poorly, his appetite usually plummets and he'll most likely want to revert to cuddles and milk feeds. Don't despair. It's like anything – feeding and sleeping routines go out of the window, but normal activity is resumed as soon as he's feeling better. As much as I hate any of mine being poorly, and would sooner it was me every time, I love all the snuggly comforting cuddle time that comes with it, as it happens less and less the more independent they all become, so enjoy it while it lasts.

If you're finding that your baby just isn't that interested in food, it could be something as simple as having too much milk. Don't starve them before a feed, but pick a mealtime where he's not too tired and hasn't got a completely empty stomach, and try him with some solids then. So long as he's got water to quench his thirst alongside the food, he'll hopefully be open to trying more solids. You've always got the bottle or breast to offer once his interest wanes but only when you feel like he's had a good go.

HOW TO START

On that first momentous day of weaning onto solids, I always found breakfast to be the best time to start. You will have been up since the crack of dawn no doubt, so make sure your baby has had his usual milk feed. This way, he won't be starving when he first tries to feed himself. Not much food will reach his tummy in the early days.

Make sure you have safeguarded as large an area of the floor as you can manage around your little self-feeder. When you start, you can't possibly imagine the mess that one baby can make with two relatively inoffensive items such as a banana and a rice cake. It will go everywhere. There's a lot to be said for giving birth to a winter baby so the baby-led weaning process starts in the warm summer months, when you can strip him down to a nappy and hose down the high chair and patio afterwards – and your baby too!!

Get yourself a cuppa and your baby a free-flow spout beaker of tap water. Start by offering him some cooked veggies – try and give him a couple of options so he realizes he's being given a choice, an actual say in what he eats, how much he eats and the freedom to play with and discard it if he doesn't much fancy swallowing any of it today. The key – particularly in the first few weeks, while he learns that it's just as fun to eat the food as it is to play with it – is to let him have fun exploring foods for himself. Imagine the excitement he'll feel squeezing that juicy pear in his fist until all the sweet juice trickles out, before wiping it all over his face in an attempt to eat it.

Definitely have your phone on hand to capture those first taste moments: the grimacing, the shock and delight on his face when he bites the end off something and moves it around his mouth as awkwardly as a cow chewing the cud. Toys don't taste this good!

On the other hand, if your baby isn't the slightest bit interested and immediately throws both foods on the floor, then don't push it. Try again next mealtime. Be completely guided by him. He'll let you know when he's ready and what he does and doesn't want to eat. So long as you're offering a variety of healthy foods, you're doing it right!

Finally, at the end of every meal just do a quick 'all clear' check of his mouth to make sure nothing's got stuck anywhere. I can remember my friend Lucy's baby gurning madly after he'd finished his finger of buttered bread, and it was only when she checked that she discovered the majority of it glued to the roof of his mouth. The poor thing had no chance of dislodging it by himself – the more he sucked, the more strongly it stuck!

FIRST FOODS

It's as simple as this. If it's not on the list of restricted foods on pages 18–21, if it's got a soft texture when raw or can be cooked to tenderize, and you've cut it into sticks or strips so your baby can hold it, then it's fine to use! If you're giving your baby something he can feed himself with a spoon, it needs to be a sticky meal, so that it sticks to the spoon without him having to try too hard when he stabs at the bowl! Things like porridge and mashed potato work well. These are some good first foods to start with:

Raw vegetables:	Cucumber, peppers, tomatoes, avocado
Cooked fruit:	Apple, pear, peach
Raw fruit:	Banana, mango, papaya, orange, kiwi fruit, ripe pear
Starchy foods:	Oats, pearl barley, rice, potatoes, quinoa, semolina
Meat, fish and other protein-rich foods:	Chicken, beef, lamb, white fish, salmon, eggs, soya beans, lentils, chickpeas
Full-fat dairy foods:	Cream cheese, mild hard cheese, plain live yoghurt or Greek yoghurt, unsalted butter, cottage cheese

MONTH-BY-MONTH PLAN

6 MONTHS

At this early stage, your baby will consume very little food, but so long as he's interested and enjoying the experience, that's what you want. Don't feel you need to do three meals a day. This whole process depends on how your baby reacts. Be completely guided by him, and don't rush it. You might spend the first couple of weaning weeks with only one successful mealtime. Every baby is different, so there's no one-size-fits-all schedule for this.

7 MONTHS

At seven months, just continue doing what you're doing. With every day that passes, your baby's mouth muscles, resolve and aim(!) will be getting stronger. At seven months, trying to push fistfuls of food into his mouth and keeping it in is still the name of the game. If you pre-load a spoon with food and give it to him to hold, he'll be trying his best to copy other diners and get it into his mouth. Try to ensure he's getting a good balance of nutrients from the foods you're giving him. At seven months, strips of meat are great for topping up his protein quota.

If you've been feeding your baby in a Bumbo-type chair up to now, it's probably time to move him into a high chair (see page 27). This will feel like progress to both of you and we all enjoy a change of scene. You might find there are some teeth coming through, though this won't make much of a difference until the back teeth appear much later on. Apart from being able to bite the end of a finger of food more successfully, your baby still lacks the ability to eat trickier foods like the hard peel on apples, particularly if he has literally bitten off more than he can chew! So keep to soft foods for the moment. Having said that, there is super-human strength in those gums and they are not to be underestimated!

Hopefully you're not too fed up with the mess. Rest assured, it won't always be this full on! Especially as your baby gets better at eating and more food ends up in his tummy than on the floor – although if he's not keen on a particular flavour, he'll probably want to get that as far away from his tray table as possible.

You might start to see your baby becoming a little more dexterous in terms of grabbing food. The grasp reflex with which babies are born with starts to diminish around this age, meaning they realize they can open a fist as well as clench it shut. So you might see some food swapping from hand to hand as he practises that. Mastering the pincer grip is the biggest milestone – the one that will make the greatest difference to feeding. But you might have to wait a few more weeks before you see that.

8 MONTHS

By month eight, you should have a much more proficient little self-feeder on your hands. There might not be such a need for you to turn every food into a soft stick – particularly if the pincer grip has been mastered, allowing your baby to pick up things between thumb and index finger rather than with the fist grab he's being using up until now.

There will still be a regular amount of gagging as your baby learns to chew and attempt to swallow, which is all normal. If you're getting him weighed regularly, you might find his weight hasn't gone up much since you started, but this will change as he gets better at self-feeding.

By eight months, your little one will most likely be hungry for two meals a day, if not three. You'll definitely have noticed a drop in the need for milk, and he might even have dropped one of the daytime milk feeds altogether. After I started weaning, the first mid-morning feed was the first to go with all of my children. Once your baby's getting a good breakfast, lunch and/or dinner, he will have less room for milk. Don't drop the milk feeds altogether, though! It's still important to ensure your baby is receiving the minimum milk requirement for his age.

A sure-fire way of being able to assess how well your baby is getting on, if you still can't make out from the mess in the kitchen how much food has actually reached his tummy, is from his nappies. If food starts going in, you'll soon start to see evidence of it in his nappy, and as gross as that sounds it will be a comfort to know baby-led weaning is working! Beware of foods that may affect the colour of what's in his nappy. You'll know what I mean if you've ever given your baby beetroot! Before you panic, try to remember what he's eaten in the last day or two. In most cases, you'll be reassured, but always check with your GP or health visitor if you are unsure.

By the end of nine months, the all-important pincer grip should be fully active, allowing your baby to pick up smaller foods. And it's this, combined with all that chewing and swallowing they've been practising up until now, that suddenly means more food ends up in his tummy than on the floor, you and the walls. Hurrah! I hear you cry. It's very welcome to see it all coming together. Success breeds confidence and vice versa, so there will be no stopping your little self-feeder once this stage has been reached. Talking of active, your baby is probably extremely mobile by now and whether he's crawling or walking, he will be burning up more energy than ever, so it's important to keep him well fuelled, but best not reach for the biscuit tin! Just like the rest of us, babies need lots of foods that release energy slowly. Complex carbohydrates such as pulses, oats and whole grains are good examples. You're probably doing three meals a day by now and perhaps even a few snacks in between or when you're out and about. This is all great stuff, so well done, you, for persevering! Over the coming months, just continue doing what you're doing. Make sure you're still offering new foods. Life's so busy, it can be easy to find yourself making the same old recipes, with the same ingredients. It's not to say you need to seek out and cook from a whole new range of dishes – just when you have time, see if there's anything new you haven't tried with your dexterous little weaning expert. You can continue to challenge your baby at mealtimes and not just with what he's eating. Yes, the time has come for DINNERWARE! All this time, you've both probably preferred to have foods laid out directly on the tray table, which has worked well. But the time will come when you should introduce a bowl or a plate, and even a fork and spoon, into the mix. Be patient with the cutlery – typically babies won't be able to use it effectively until around 12 months!

Children learn best by example, so the more you seat them at the table to eat with the rest of the family – who are all hopefully pretty skilled with dinnerware and cutlery! – the quicker they'll pick it up. It will take time, and you will end up with things clattering to the floor, but the sooner you get your baby used to it, the better. Just think: you'll be able to eat out in a restaurant, without having to clean the floor before you leave, if you can train him to keep it on the plate. This is when bowls with suckers that stick to the table are a godsend. Your baby will soon learn that his bowl isn't going anywhere. An added bonus is that you can start serving sloppy, runny meals like soup, increasing the range of options to serve for supper in the process.

BABY CEREAL PANCAKES

Makes about 13 pancakes | ❄ *Suitable for freezing*

I'm all for eating up leftovers and these small American-style pancakes are
a perfect way to use up leftover porridge – such as the Carrot and Apricot
Porridge on page 86 – and boost its nutritional value at the same time. Finger
foods are important as they help your child to develop his pincer grip, learn how
to feed himself and also to develop the jaw muscles needed for speech.

1 ripe banana, peeled and
   chopped

100g/3½g self-raising flour

½ tsp ground cinnamon

1 egg, lightly beaten

100ml/3½fl oz full-fat milk

75g/3oz ready-cooked thick
   porridge, cooled

Unsalted butter or sunflower
   oil, for cooking

To serve

Plain full-fat live yoghurt

Fruit compote (such as any
   of the fruit purées on pages
   58–61) or fresh fruit

1. Put the banana, flour, cinnamon, egg and milk in
   a blender and blend to a smooth batter. Stir in the
   cooked porridge and leave the batter to rest for
   20 minutes.
2. Heat enough butter or oil to coat the base of a
   large frying pan. Place 2 tablespoons of batter per
   pancake into the pan and cook over a medium heat
   for 2 minutes on each side or until set and golden.
   You can probably cook about four pancakes in the
   pan at a time.
3. Place the cooked pancakes on kitchen paper and keep
   warm on a plate in a low oven while you cook the
   remaining pancakes. Serve plain or with yoghurt, fruit
   compote or fresh fruit.

ROASTED CARROT HUMMUS

Serves about 6 (young children)

If the oven's already on, you could make the most of the heat and roast some carrots for making this hummus. Tahini is a good source of calcium, especially if your child does not like dairy products or is vegan. Serve the dip with pitta bread, cut into fingers, and vegetable sticks (steamed first, if giving to young babies).

275g/10oz carrots, scrubbed/peeled, quartered lengthways and cut into batons

1 tbsp extra-virgin olive oil, plus extra for drizzling

1 tbsp tahini

4–5 tbsp coconut drinking milk (from a carton)

1–2 tsp lemon juice

1. Preheat the oven to 190°C/375°F/Gas 5.
2. Toss the carrots in a little of the olive oil until lightly coated. Spread them out on a baking tray and roast in the oven for 25–30 minutes, turning once, until tender and starting to turn golden.
3. Tip the roasted carrots into a food processor or use a hand blender. Add the 1 tablespoon of olive oil, tahini and the smaller amount of coconut milk and lemon juice. Blend until smooth and creamy, then taste and add the remaining coconut milk or lemon juice, if needed.
4. Spoon the hummus into a bowl and either serve straight away or keep in an airtight container in the fridge for up to three days.

» Roasting intensifies the flavour and sweetness of the carrots as well as increasing the availability of vitamin A – essential for healthy vision and skin.

SEEDY BREADSTICKS

Makes about 15 breadsticks | ✳ *Suitable for freezing (uncooked or cooked)*

They may be small and unassuming, but seeds are bursting with nutrients, including bone-healthy magnesium, copper and zinc. These pimped-up soft breadsticks make a tasty snack, whether eaten plain or dunked into a dip. If you want to crisp them up, bake them for 15–20 minutes longer, at 130°C/250°F/Gas ½, after the main cooking time.

2 tbsp mixed seeds (such as sunflower, pumpkin and poppy)

250g/9oz mix of wholemeal and white bread flour, plus extra if needed and for dusting

1 tsp fast-action dried yeast

1 tsp sea salt

1 tbsp ground flaxseeds/linseeds

1 tsp honey or maple syrup

160ml/5½fl oz lukewarm water, plus extra if needed

1½ tbsp olive oil, plus extra for greasing

1. Place the mixed seeds in a spice/coffee grinder or food processor and grind to a coarse powder, then set aside.

2. In a large bowl, mix together the flour, yeast, salt, flaxseeds, honey or maple syrup and the freshly ground seeds. Add the water and olive oil, then mix initially with a wooden spoon and then with your fingers to make a soft, slightly sticky dough, adding more water or flour if the dough seems either too dry or too wet.

3. Dust a worktop with flour and knead the dough for 10 minutes. Push the dough flat with the palm of your hand, fold the far edge over towards you and give it a half turn, then repeat. Place the dough in a clean bowl, cover with cling film and leave in a warm place for 30 minutes or until slightly risen.

4. Divide the dough into 15 pieces (about 30g/1¼oz each). Lightly grease your hands with a little olive oil and roll one piece of dough into a long, thin sausage shape. Repeat with the remaining dough, to make about 15 breadsticks in total. Place the breadsticks on two lightly greased baking sheets, cover with cling film and leave to rest for 15 minutes.

5. Meanwhile, preheat the oven to 200°C/400°F/Gas 6.

6. Brush the breadsticks with a little extra oil and bake in the oven for 15–20 minutes or until risen and lightly golden. Transfer to a wire rack to cool. You can store them in an airtight container for up to three days.

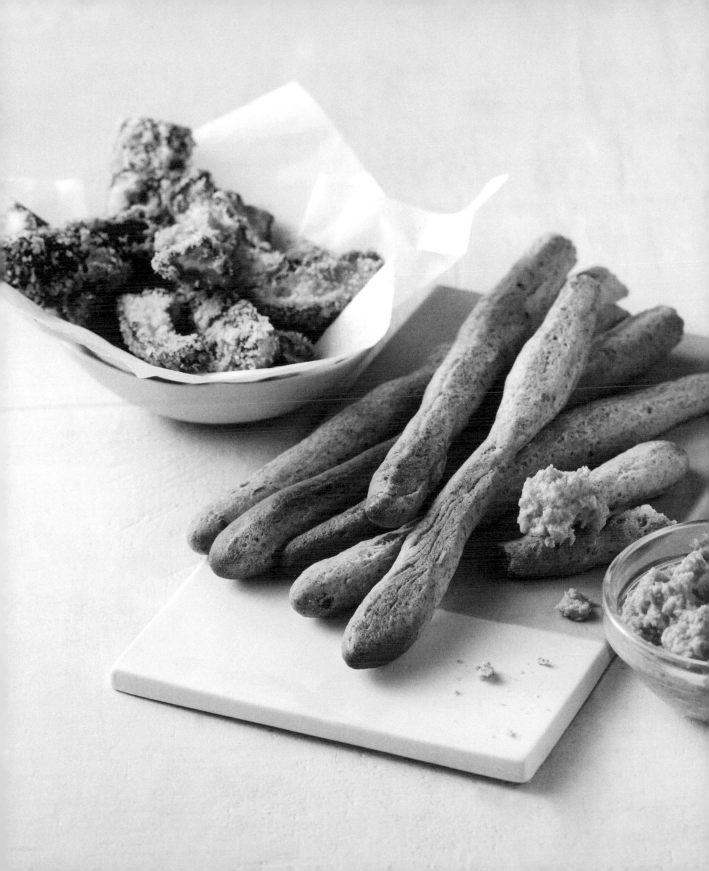

CHEESY CAULI AND COURGETTE CHIPS

Serves 4 (young children)

The crisp and golden cheesy coating covering these cauliflower florets and courgette sticks makes them a whole lot more interesting, and it's another way to encourage your little one to eat more veg. Broccoli florets also taste great prepared this way.

Olive oil, for greasing

4 tbsp ground almonds

40g/1½oz finely grated Parmesan cheese

2 eggs

2 good-sized courgettes, cut into thirds and each third quartered lengthways

125g/4½oz small cauliflower florets

1. Preheat the oven to 190°C/375°F/Gas 5 and grease a large baking tray with olive oil.
2. Mix together the ground almonds and Parmesan in a shallow bowl. Beat the eggs in a separate bowl.
3. Dunk each courgette stick and cauliflower floret briefly into the beaten egg and then the ground almond mixture until lightly coated all over. Place on the oiled baking tray in a single, evenly spaced layer.
4. Roast in the oven for 20–25 minutes or until the cheesy coating is crisp and golden and the vegetables are tender. Leave to cool slightly before serving as a finger food or side dish.

ROASTED RED PEPPER DIP

Serves about 4 (young children)

A cinch to make – just bung all the ingredients in a blender and blitz until smooth. As raw garlic can be a bit strong for babies, it is lightly simmered in the olive oil first to calm its pungency. Serve the dip in small bowls with fingers of pitta bread and vegetable sticks (steamed first, if giving to young babies), or the Seedy Breadsticks on page 198, for a quick lunch or snack.

3 tbsp olive oil

1 large garlic clove, peeled and cut in half

60g/2½oz roasted red peppers in oil, drained

40g/1½oz fresh breadcrumbs

1 tbsp ground almonds

Juice of ½ lemon

Put the olive oil and garlic in a small saucepan and warm gently for 2 minutes. Pour the garlic-infused oil into a food processor, or use a hand blender, and add the rest of the ingredients. Blitz to a fairly smooth paste, adding a splash of boiled water for a looser consistency. If not using straight away, store in the fridge in an airtight container for up to three days.

SMOKED MACKEREL HUMMUS

Serves about 6 (young children)

The strong flavour of smoked mackerel can be off-putting for young ones, but mix the omega-3-rich fish with plain yoghurt and chickpeas, and you tame any fishiness, without losing any of the health benefits. Serve with steamed vegetable sticks (for young children) and pitta bread fingers for dunking.

100g/3½oz smoked mackerel fillets, skin and pin bones removed

50g/2oz plain full-fat live yoghurt

100g/3½oz tinned chickpeas, drained and rinsed

Juice of ½ lemon

Cut the fish into large pieces and place in a food processor or use a hand blender. Add the yoghurt, chickpeas and lemon, and blend until smooth and creamy. Spoon the hummus into a bowl and serve straight away or keep in an airtight container in the fridge for up to two days.

BAKED FALAFEL BALLS

Makes about 15 falafel balls | ❄ *Suitable for freezing (uncooked or cooked)*

These little balls of goodness are very adaptable – serve them hot or cold on their own or with a pot of hummus (see pages 197 and 201) or the Roasted Red Pepper Dip on page 201. They're also delicious stuffed into a pitta bread or wrapped in a Little Gem lettuce leaf.

400g/14oz tin of chickpeas, drained and rinsed

2 large garlic cloves, peeled

1 raw beetroot (about 75g/3oz), peeled and roughly chopped

1 tsp dried mint

2 tsp ground coriander

1 tsp turmeric

1½ tbsp plain flour

Olive oil, for brushing

2 tbsp sesame seeds (optional)

1. Preheat the oven to 190°C/375°F/Gas 5 and line a baking tray with baking paper.
2. Put the chickpeas, garlic and beetroot in a food processor and blitz to a coarse paste. Spoon the mixture into a large bowl and stir in the mint, ground spices and the flour – the paste will be fairly wet but should hold together when pressed into small balls.
3. With damp hands, form the mixture into balls, each about the size of a walnut. Brush each falafel with oil, then dunk into the sesame seeds (if using), until lightly coated. Repeat with the remaining falafel mixture to make about 15 in total. Bake in the oven for 25–30 minutes or until golden and firm.

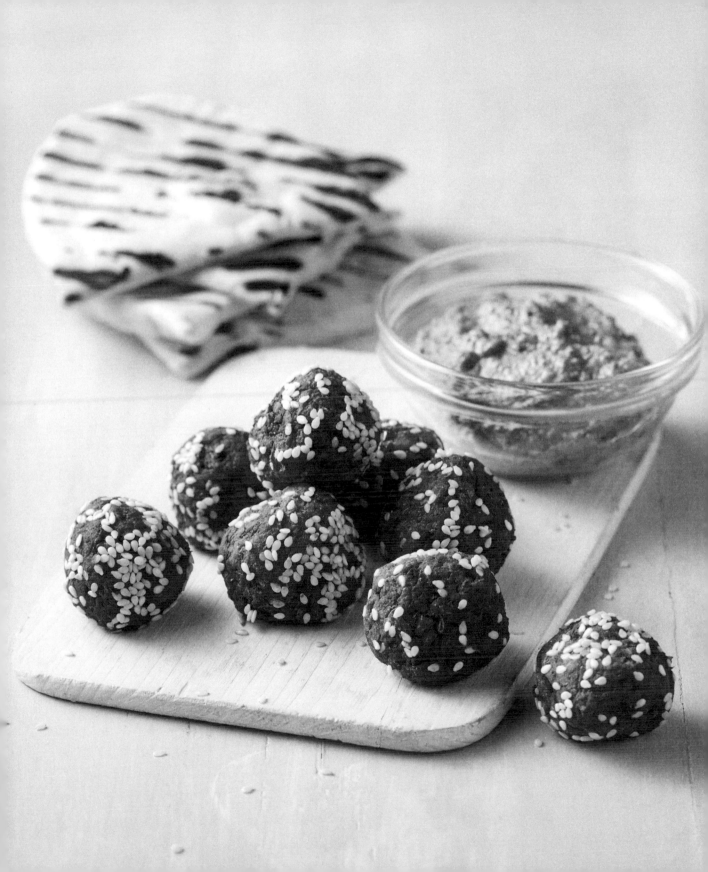

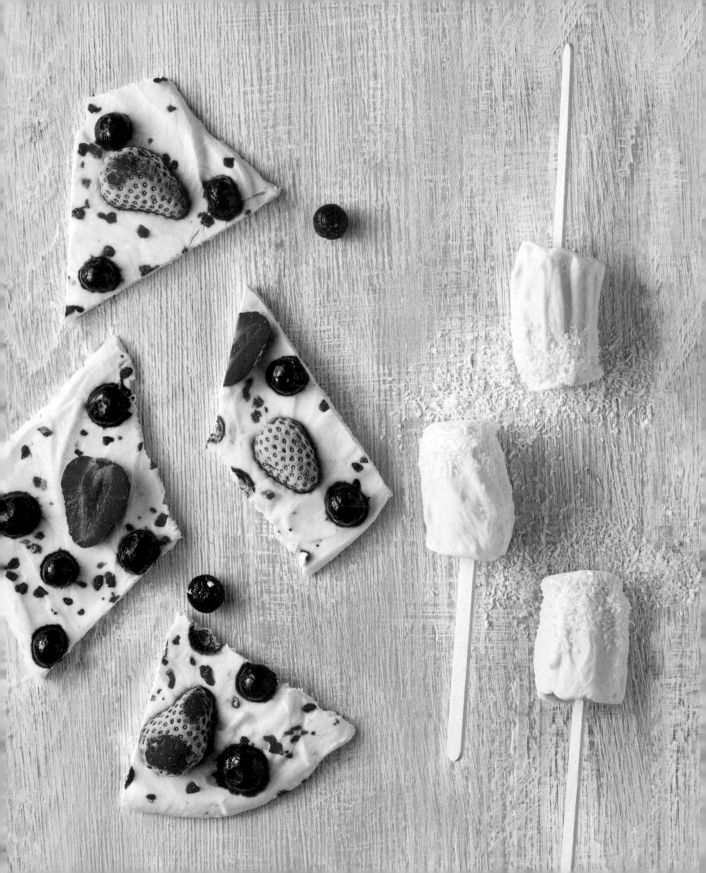

FRUITY YOGHURT FINGERS

Makes about 10 fingers | ✳ Suitable for freezing

A delicious cooling, fruity treat that takes next to no time to prepare and is perfect for soothing teething pain. I've suggested a few fruit toppings, but do choose your own favourites and see below for more ideas. For babies under one year, leave out the maple syrup or honey and mash or purée the fruit before stirring it into the yoghurt.

250g/9oz plain full-fat live Greek yoghurt

1 teaspoon vanilla extract

1 tablespoon maple syrup or honey (optional)

60g/2½oz frozen blueberries

60g/2½oz strawberries, hulled and halved or quartered if large

2 tbsp freeze-dried raspberries or strawberries

1. Pour the yoghurt into a large bowl and stir in the vanilla extract and maple syrup or honey (if using).
2. Line a large baking tray with baking paper. Tip the yoghurt mixture on to the tray and spread out to a long rectangle, about 10 x 20cm/4 x 8in and 1cm/½in thick. Scatter the blueberries, strawberries and freeze-dried berries over the top, pressing them down slightly into the yoghurt mix. Cover the tray with cling film and freeze for 1¾ hours or until almost frozen.
3. Remove the frozen yoghurt from the freezer and cut into about ten fingers, then return to the freezer and leave until firm. Take as many yoghurt fingers as you need out of the freezer 15 minutes before serving to soften slightly. Store the remaining fingers in a freezer-proof container or bag for up to two months.

More topping ideas

Swap the blueberries, strawberries and freeze-dried berries in the recipe above for a similar quantity of one or more of the following:

* Small chunks of fresh mango, kiwi, peach or banana
* Fresh or frozen raspberries, blackcurrants or blackberries
* Dried fruit (such as raisins, sour cherries, cranberries or chopped apricots/dates)
* Granola (see pages 118 and 152)
* Unsweetened desiccated coconut
* Chopped nuts (such as pecans, hazelnuts or almonds)
* Chocolate drops

FROZEN BANANA POPS

Makes 6 ice lollies | ❄ *Suitable for freezing*

These yoghurt-coated banana lollies are a great simple treat. If you're making them for a baby under the age of one, do leave out the maple syrup or honey (ripe bananas may be sweet enough already) and, it goes without saying, keep an eye on young children while they are eating a lolly to avoid any risk of choking on the stick. No lolly sticks? Instead, freeze the bananas and blend with the yoghurt mix for a delicious ice cream.

150g/5oz plain full-fat live Greek yoghurt

1 tsp vanilla extract

1 tbsp maple syrup or honey (optional)

3 tbsp unsweetened desiccated coconut (optional)

2 large just-ripe bananas, peeled and each one cut into thirds

You will need 6 lolly sticks

1. Line a small baking tray with baking paper. Mix together the yoghurt, vanilla extract and maple syrup or honey (if using) in a small bowl. Put the desiccated coconut (if using) in a separate small bowl.
2. Insert a lolly stick into one end of each banana chunk. Holding the stick, dunk each banana chunk into the yoghurt mix to evenly coat, and then dip the top end into the coconut.
3. Place the coated banana chunks, sticks pointing upwards, on the lined baking tray and freeze for 3 hours or until firm. When frozen, transfer the banana pops to a freezer bag until ready to eat.

Yoghurt drops

If you have any leftover yoghurt, spoon it in peaked blobs on a baking tray lined with baking paper and freeze until firm. Transfer to a freezer-proof container or bag and store for up to two months. Serve the frozen yoghurt drops as finger food or allow to soften slightly and then serve in a bowl.

NO-ADDED-SUGAR TEETHING BISCUITS

Makes about 14 biscuits | ✳ *Suitable for freezing (uncooked)*

A doddle to make, these biscuits should bring some relief, I hope, to dreaded teething pain and they are naturally sweetened with banana, rather than added sugar. It goes without saying that you should not leave your child alone when eating, particularly when it comes to foods such as rice cakes, rusks and teething biscuits, which can crumble or break up and hence pose a choking risk.

Sunflower oil, for greasing

100g/3½oz rolled porridge oats

125g/4½oz self-raising flour

½ tsp ground cinnamon (optional)

4 tbsp mashed ripe banana or other thick fruit purée (see pages 60–1)

1 egg, lightly beaten

1 tsp vanilla extract

1. Preheat the oven to 180°C/350°F/Gas 4 and lightly grease a large baking sheet with a little sunflower oil.
2. Blitz the oats in a food processor until finely ground, then tip them into a large bowl with the flour and the cinnamon (if using).
3. Beat together the banana, egg and vanilla extract. Stir the banana mixture into the flour mixture, first with a fork and then using your hands, until it comes together into a stiff dough. Lightly knead the dough into smooth ball.
4. Divide the dough into 14 pieces and form each piece into a rectangular biscuit, about 1cm/½in thick and 2cm/¾in wide and with rounded edges. Place on the prepared baking sheet and bake in the oven for 30–35 minutes or until golden and crisp. Leave to cool on a wire rack and store in an airtight container for up to five days; they will soften slightly with time but still taste good.

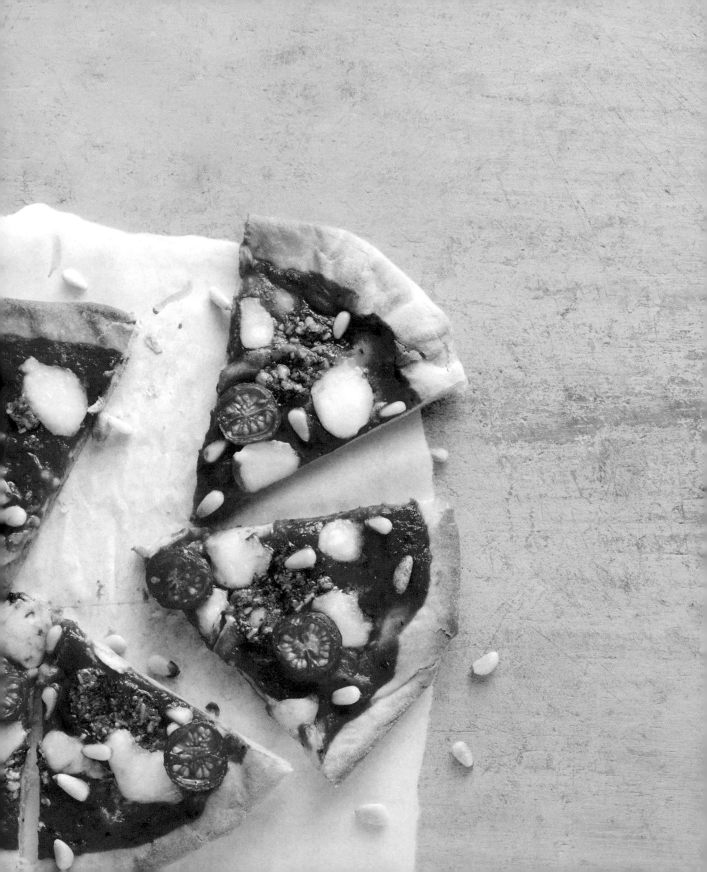

Chapter 6

15 MONTHS AND BEYOND

Many parents notice increased fussiness when it comes to food at this age, typically because their little one is becoming more single-minded and trying to assert her independence. Despite this, from 15 months your job is to make sure you're still offering your child a varied and nutritionally balanced meal three times a day, with healthy snacks in between. Hopefully, they'll be more accustomed to a variety of flavours and textures by now, so you can have a bit more fun with meals. Breakfast, lunch and dinner really start to resemble what you have on your own plate.

HOW MUCH TO FEED YOUR TODDLER

Your toddler might (if you're lucky!) be getting to grips with cutlery by now, which gives you the perfect opportunity to start letting them listen to their instincts when it comes to portion control. With the independence of feeding themselves (albeit with a little help from Mum or Dad now and again) comes the independence of acknowledging and responding to their own needs.

PORTION SIZE

At this age, your little one might be embracing all sorts of textures but the key thing to remember is that mealtimes should be served in an approachable way. If you're serving your toddler a Quick Pan Pizza (see page 224), for example, make sure it's cut up into bite-sized pieces so she's not overwhelmed! As ever, every baby is different and, depending on what she's eaten that day, will be able to manage different amounts of food at different meals.

If you're serving up nutritious meals and your baby is a healthy weight, you don't need to worry too much about whether she's finishing everything on her plate. As with the 12–15-month stage, be careful to monitor how many snacks she's eating throughout the day. I know it can be really tempting to throw snacks at your toddler in a bid to keep her occupied while you get some chores done, but there's nothing more frustrating than when you've lovingly prepared dinner for the family only to find that she has zero appetite.

By this stage, the bottle is hopefully a distant memory. Nonetheless, milk is still an important part of your baby's diet, whether breast or dairy. So even though she might be much more interested in the delicious solids she's getting to grips with, make sure you still supplement her diet with milk.

SAMPLE MENU

Breakfast — Apple Wholewheat Muesli (see page 213)

Mid-morning — Baby's usual milk feed, and Cheesy Cauli and Courgette Chips (see page 200) or cucumber sticks with Roasted Red Pepper Dip (see page 201) as a nutritious snack

Lunch — Mexican Scramble Wrap (see page 220)

Mid-afternoon — Toast fingers spread with some Mixed Nut Butter (see page 280)

Teatime — Weekday Chicken Roast (see page 230) or Best Veggie Burgers (see page 221), for the whole family, followed by Easiest Banana Pudding Ever (see page 241)

Bedtime — Baby's usual milk feed

START-THE-DAY SMOOTHIE

Serves 2 (1 young child + 1 adult)

If your child is not a big eater first thing, then a thick and protein-rich smoothie can be good way to pack in a few extra nutrients. Just bear in mind that it's not intended to be a complete meal but as a supplement to other breakfast foods.

2 bananas, peeled

1 rounded tsp smooth peanut butter or other nut butter (for homemade see page 280)

½ tsp ground flaxseeds/linseeds

300ml/11fl oz full-fat milk

100g/3½ oz plain full-fat live yoghurt

¼ tsp ground cinnamon

Put all the ingredients in a blender and blend until smooth and creamy – adding a splash more milk if it's too thick.

IMMUNE-BOOST JUICE

Serves 2 (1 young child + 1 adult)

A new term at school or nursery often brings with it all sorts of bugs, and this vitamin C-loaded juice helps to boost the immune system and fight off colds. The juice is diluted with water to curb the sweetness and acidity of the fruit and help protect the teeth. To reduce the risk of tooth decay, it would be best to give it as part of a meal.

Flesh of 1 small ripe mango, roughly chopped

Freshly squeezed juice of 2 oranges

¼ tsp finely grated fresh root ginger

Squeeze of lemon juice

Put all the ingredients in a blender and blend until smooth. Pour in enough water to double the quantity of liquid – it should be 50 per cent fruit purée and 50 per cent water – and blend again.

APPLE WHOLEWHEAT MUESLI

Serves 4 (2 young children + 2 adults)

Made with wheat or oat flakes, this is a healthy twist on regular muesli. Serve with milk and a few blueberries or other pieces of fresh fruit scattered on top.

100g/3½oz wholewheat or oat flakes

12 pecan halves, chopped

4 tbsp sunflower seeds

4 tsp ground flaxseeds/linseeds

½ tsp ground cinnamon

60g/2½oz dried apple slices, or other dried fruit, finely chopped

1. Combine all the ingredients in a large bowl.
2. Store in an airtight container for up to a week. For a finer-textured muesli, blitz in a food processor, then stir in the finely chopped apple or other dried fruit just before serving.

BREAKFAST ENERGY BALLS

Makes 12 balls

These are full of energy. Serve one as a precursor to savoury foods, such as a boiled egg and soldiers, for a complete breakfast.

3 heaped tbsp jumbo porridge oats

1 small carrot scrubbed/peeled and roughly chopped

100g/3½oz pitted dates, chopped

1 rounded tsp nut butter (see page 280)

3 tbsp ground almonds

1 tbsp cocoa or cacao powder

½ tsp chia seeds (optional)

25g/1oz desiccated coconut and/or extra cocoa/cacao powder, for dusting

1. Put the oats and carrot in a food processor and process until finely chopped. Add the dates and nut butter, and process again to a smooth paste, occasionally scraping down the sides of the processor bowl, if needed, to ensure the mixture is evenly blended. Stir in the ground almonds, cocoa or cacao powder and the chia seeds (if using) to make a thick paste.
2. Sprinkle the desiccated coconut and/or cocoa/cacao powder on separate plates.
3. Shape the oat mixture into 12 walnut-sized balls and roll them in the desiccated coconut or the cocoa/cacao powder until lightly coated. They will keep in an airtight pot in the fridge for up to two weeks.

VANILLA FRENCH TOAST WITH QUICK STRAWBERRY JAM

Serves 4 (2 young children + 2 adults)

This twist on savoury eggy bread comes with a no-added-sugar instant jam made with fresh strawberries, though you could substitute with a fruit purée (see pages 60–1) or, if you're short on time, with a shop-bought low-sugar jam. For little ones, cut the French toast into fingers for dunking into the jam.

2 eggs, lightly beaten

3 tbsp full-fat milk

1 tsp vanilla extract

½ tsp ground cinnamon

4 thick slices of wholemeal bread (or brioche for a treat)

25g/1oz unsalted butter

Thick plain full-fat live yoghurt, to serve

For the quick strawberry jam

175g/6oz strawberries, hulled

2 tsp chia seeds (preferably white)

1 tsp vanilla extract

Squeeze of lemon juice

1. First make the quick strawberry jam. Purée half the fruit using a hand blender and stir in the chia seeds. Leave for 30 minutes, stirring occasionally, or until the seeds swell and the purée thickens. Using the back of a fork, roughly mash the rest of the strawberries and stir in the vanilla extract and lemon juice. Stir the chia mixture into the mashed strawberries and set aside to thicken further to a jam-like consistency.

2. Mix together the eggs, milk, vanilla extract and cinnamon in a shallow bowl. Add two slices of the bread, pressing them down to immerse them in the egg mixture.

3. Melt half the butter in a large frying pan over a medium-low heat. Add the egg-soaked bread and fry for 2–3 minutes on each side or until golden. While the bread is cooking, add the remaining two slices to the remaining egg mixture to soak.

4. Remove the French toast from the pan and serve straight away or keep warm in a low oven while you cook the remaining bread in the rest of the butter. Serve with a spoonful of the jam and a dollop of yoghurt.

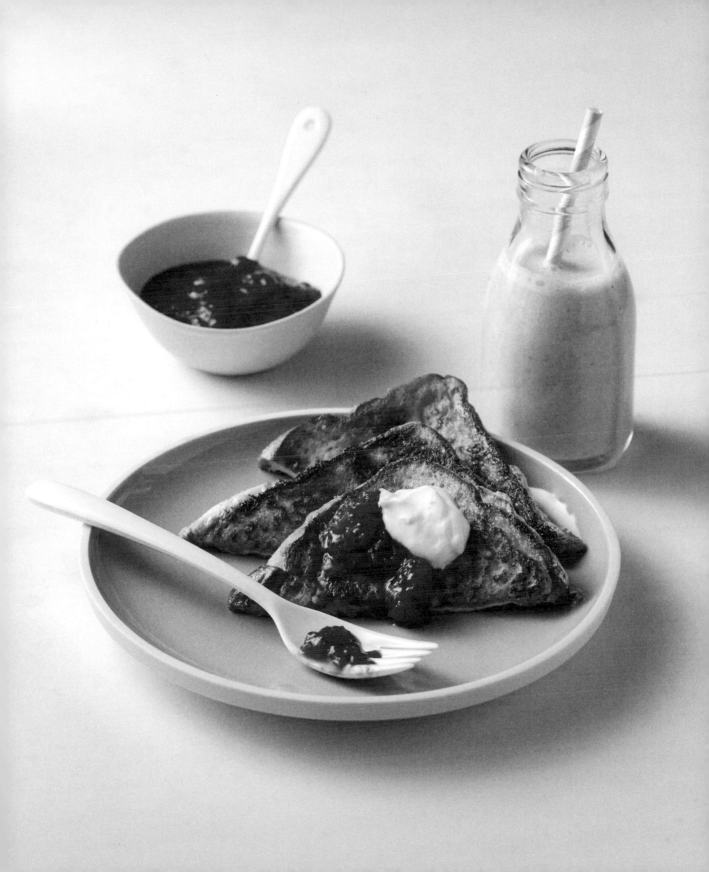

BAKED EGG CUPS

Serves 4 (2 young children + 2 adults)

Health-wise, eggs are amazing: they're an excellent, inexpensive source of high-quality protein, vitamins, minerals and good fats. They're also incredibly versatile and super-easy to prepare. Here, they are baked in a ramekin with cheese and spinach.

15g/½oz butter, cut into small pieces, plus extra for greasing

4 eggs

20g/¾oz mature Cheddar cheese, grated

4 tbsp full-fat milk

20g/¾oz baby leaf spinach, finely chopped

2 small tomatoes, halved and deseeded

Freshly ground black pepper

Wholegrain seedy bread, toasted, to serve

You will need 4 ramekins or similar-sized small ovenproof dishes

1. Preheat the oven to 180°C/350°F/Gas 4 and lightly grease the ramekins with butter.
2. Beat together the eggs, cheese, milk and spinach in a jug, season with black pepper then pour the mixture into the prepared ramekins.
3. Place the ramekins in a small roasting tin and pour in enough just-boiled water to come halfway up the sides of the ramekins. This helps the eggs to cook evenly all the way through. Top each one with a tomato half and dot over the butter.
4. Place in the oven and bake for 17–20 minutes or until just set. Carefully remove the roasting tin from the oven, take out the ramekins and leave to cool slightly. For young children, scoop the egg mixture into a bowl and chop. Serve with the toast.

GOLD STAR SOUP

Serves 6 (4 young children + 2 adults) | ✽ *Suitable for freezing*

Abundant in vitamins and minerals, this substantial smooth golden soup makes a filling lunch or supper with crusty bread.

1 tbsp olive oil

1 large onion, chopped

400g/14oz carrots, scrubbed/ peeled and chopped

300g/11oz butternut squash, peeled, deseeded and cut into chunks

60g/2½oz split red lentils, rinsed

2 garlic cloves, finely chopped

1cm/½in piece of fresh root ginger, grated (no need to peel)

1 tsp ground turmeric

1 litre/1¾ pints salt-free vegetable stock (for homemade stock, see page 109)

Good squeeze of lemon juice

Freshly ground black pepper

Crusty bread, to serve

1. Heat the olive oil in a large saucepan over a medium heat, add the onion and cook for 5 minutes, stirring frequently, until softened.
2. Add the carrots, squash, lentils, garlic, ginger, turmeric and stock, then bring almost to the boil. Turn down the heat slightly and simmer, partially covered with a lid, for 25 minutes or until the lentils and vegetables are tender.
3. Blitz the soup until smooth using a blender or hand-held blender, then stir in the lemon juice and add a grind of black pepper. Serve with crusty bread.

» Research shows turmeric can help improve our memory and, interestingly, black pepper has been shown to help the body absorb it properly.

WATERMELON SALAD STICKS WITH PITTA CRISPS

Serves 4 (2 young children + 2 adults)

Any attempt to make salad more child-friendly and fun is good with me. Here, the bite-sized chunks of fresh fruit and veg are threaded on to cocktail sticks or wooden kebab skewers, ready to be dunked into the minty yoghurt dressing. Of course, you don't have to use sticks or skewers, and definitely leave them out if serving to young children – just drizzle the dressing over.

2 wholegrain pitta breads

Olive oil, for brushing

200g/7oz watermelon, peeled, deseeded and cut into 1cm/½in chunks

100g/3½oz mozzarella (or smoked tofu or cooked chicken, ham or salmon), cut into 1cm/½in chunks

7.5cm/3in piece of cucumber, quartered, deseeded and cut into 1cm/½in chunks

40g/1½oz pitted black or green olives, cut in half

Flesh of 1 ripe avocado, cut into 1cm/½in chunks and tossed in a little lemon juice to stop it discolouring

For the minty yoghurt dip

90g/3½oz plain full-fat live yoghurt

4 tbsp very finely chopped fresh mint leaves

Juice of 1 small lemon

You will need cocktail sticks or small wooden skewers

1. Preheat the oven to 180°C/350°F/Gas 4 and make the pitta crisps.
2. Cut along the edge of one of the pitta breads, open out and divide into two pieces. Repeat with the second pitta bread, so that you have four thin halves. Lightly brush both sides of each pitta half with olive oil. Place on two baking sheets and bake in the oven for 10 minutes, turning halfway, until crisp and golden. Leave to cool, then break into large pieces.
3. While the pitta halves are baking, make the salad sticks. Thread a chunk of watermelon, mozzarella and cucumber on to one cocktail stick or skewer, followed by an olive and a piece of avocado, and place in a serving dish. Repeat until you have used up all the ingredients.
4. Mix together the ingredients for the dressing, adding a splash of warm water to loosen slightly. Pour into a serving bowl and serve with the salad sticks and pitta crisps.

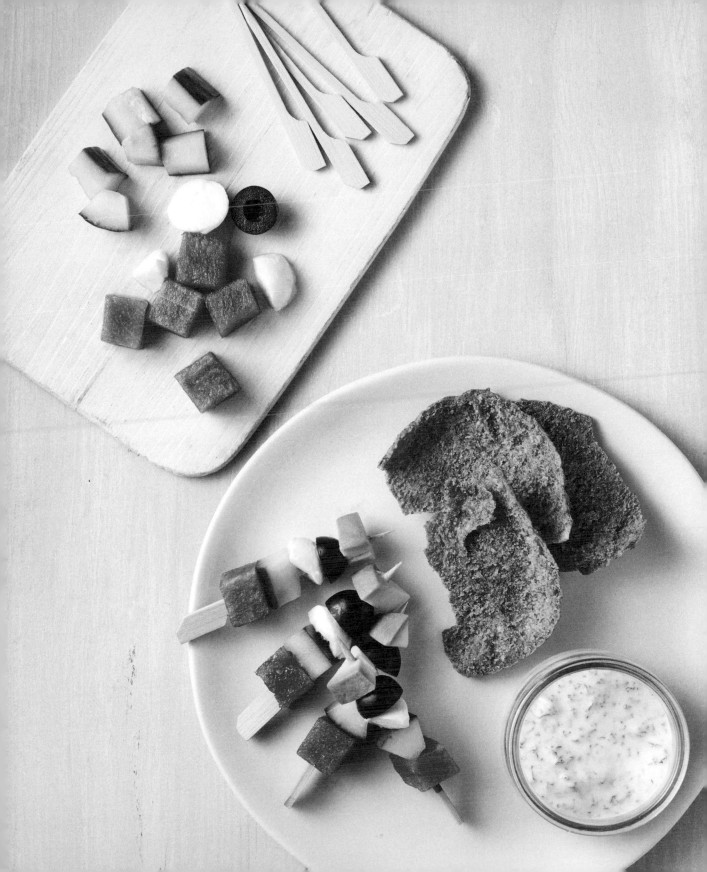

MEXICAN SCRAMBLE WRAP

Serves 2 (young children)

A take on a baked burrito, this soft floury tortilla is filled with a Mexican-inspired mix of kidney beans, avocado and scrambled egg. Young children often start to become fussy eaters around two years old, so it pays to offer plenty of variety at this age and hopefully set the tone for future food preferences. Serve the wrap with cooked or raw vegetable fingers, such as carrot, red pepper, sugar snap peas or cucumber.

2 eggs, lightly beaten

1 tbsp full-fat milk

10g/⅓oz unsalted butter

2 tbsp finely diced red pepper

4 tbsp tinned kidney beans, drained, rinsed and mashed or left whole

1 large spring onion, finely chopped

¼ tsp ground cumin

Flesh of ½ small ripe avocado, diced

1 wholemeal or corn tortilla

1. Beat together the eggs and milk in a jug and set aside.
2. Melt the butter in a small pan, add the red pepper, kidney beans and spring onion, and cook over a medium heat for 2 minutes, stirring, until softened. Add the cumin and the egg mixture, reduce the heat to medium-low and cook, gently turning the eggs until scrambled. Remove from the heat and stir in the avocado.
3. Meanwhile, heat the tortilla in a large, dry frying pan until warmed through.
4. Place the tortilla on a plate, spoon the scrambled egg mixture down one side and roll up to encase the filling, then cut in half to serve. Alternatively, cut the tortilla into wedges and serve the scrambled egg in a bowl.

BEST VEGGIE BURGERS

Makes 6 burgers | ✳ *Suitable for freezing (uncooked or cooked)*

Who needs meat when you can make veggie burgers that taste this good –
a super-nutritious blend of cooked chestnuts, pumpkin seeds, onion and
breadcrumbs. Serve the burgers in a bun with all the usual accompaniments
or with potato wedges, or shape into 'meatballs' and cook in a tomato sauce
and serve with pasta or rice.

175g/6oz pumpkin seeds

175g/6oz cooked chestnuts
(from a vacuum pack or tin),
roughly chopped

1 red onion, roughly chopped

75g/3oz day-old wholemeal
breadcrumbs

1 tsp low-salt soy sauce

2 tsp Dijon mustard

1 rounded tbsp tomato purée

1 tsp dried thyme

1 egg, lightly beaten

Sunflower oil, for cooking

Freshly ground black pepper

To serve

6 seedy burger or brioche buns,
cut in half

Green salad leaves (such as cos
or butterhead)

Tomato slices

Quick Tomato Ketchup (see
page 170)

1. Toast the pumpkin seeds in a large, dry frying pan for
   2–3 minutes, tossing the pan occasionally, until they
   start to brown. Take care as they can pop! Leave to
   cool and then grind in a food processor until finely
   chopped. Tip the chopped seeds into a large bowl.

2. Add the chestnuts to the food processor with the
   onion and process until very finely chopped. Stir
   into the pumpkin seeds with the rest of the burger
   ingredients. Season with black pepper and mix well
   to make a coarse paste – it will be quite wet but holds
   together when cooked. Using damp hands, shape the
   mixture into six burgers each about 1cm/½in thick
   and chill in the fridge for 30 minutes to firm up.

3. Heat enough oil to coat the bottom of a large frying
   pan and cook the burgers in two batches over a
   medium heat for 3 minutes on each side or until
   cooked through and golden. Serve the burgers in the
   buns, layered with salad leaves, tomato slices and a
   dollop of tomato ketchup.

NO-STIR CREAMY RISOTTO

Serves 4 (2 children + 2 adults) | ✳ *Suitable for freezing*

Risottos, however lovely, do require continuous stirring if cooked on the hob. This version, on the other hand, can be left alone to do its thing in the oven – simple! Adults may like to top the risotto with crispy pancetta or bacon – cook in the oven at the same time as the risotto until crisp, leave to cool then tear into pieces.

225g/8oz frozen peas

1 tbsp olive oil

1 large onion, roughly chopped

2 leeks, thinly sliced

75g/3oz white cabbage, finely chopped

3 garlic cloves, finely chopped

200g/7oz risotto rice

1 tsp dried thyme

800ml/25fl oz hot low-salt vegetable stock (for homemade stock, see page 109)

50g/2oz Parmesan cheese, finely grated, plus extra for serving

3 tbsp full-fat cream cheese

Good squeeze of lemon juice and 1 tbsp finely grated unwaxed zest

40g/1½oz walnut pieces (optional)

Freshly ground black pepper

1. Preheat the oven to 180°C/350°F/Gas 4. Take the peas out of the freezer and leave them to defrost.
2. Heat the oil in a large casserole dish or ovenproof saucepan, add the onion and stir-fry over a medium heat for 5 minutes. Tip in the leeks and cabbage, and cook for another 3 minutes. Stir in the garlic and rice until coated and cook for another 2 minutes. Add the thyme and stock, give everything a stir and raise the heat, heating through until the stock starts to bubble.
3. Cover the casserole dish or pan with a lid and place in the oven to cook for 20 minutes. Remove from the oven and add the peas, Parmesan, cream cheese, lemon juice and zest, and season with black pepper. Stir until everything is combined, cover and return to the oven to cook for another 5 minutes or until the peas are heated through and the rice is tender.
4. Meanwhile, lightly toast the walnut pieces (if using) in a large, dry frying pan for 2–3 minutes, tossing the pan frequently, until they smell toasted and start to brown. Leave to cool and finely chop for small children.
5. Let the risotto sit for 5 minutes out of the oven. Spoon into shallow bowls, grate over extra Parmesan and sprinkle with the toasted walnuts, if using.

» Leftover risotto can be frozen for up to a month. Don't leave the risotto at room temperature for long periods due to the risk of bacterial growth. Defrost frozen risotto in the fridge and reheat thoroughly before serving.

FISH PIZZAS

Serves 4 (2 young children + 2 adults)

If you struggle to get your child to eat fish, then this could win her over. It's so easy: white fish fillets are topped with a combination of chopped tomato, mozzarella and a sprinkling of oregano to make a sort of carb-free pizza. Why not make use of the oven and roast some potato wedges at the same time – just put them in the oven 20 minutes before the fish so they are ready to serve at the same time, along with some cooked vegetables or a salad.

Olive oil, for greasing and drizzling

4 skinless, boneless thick white fish fillets (such as cod, haddock, pollock or hake)

2 tomatoes, deseeded and finely chopped

125g/4½oz mozzarella, drained, patted dry and torn into small pieces

½ tsp dried oregano

Freshly ground black pepper

1. Preheat the oven to 180°C/350°F/Gas 4 and lightly grease a baking tray with olive oil.
2. Place the fish fillets on the baking tray. Divide the tomatoes among each fillet, spooning them evenly on top, followed by the mozzarella. Drizzle a little olive oil over the fish, sprinkle with the oregano and season with pepper.
3. Roast the fish in the oven for 20 minutes or until cooked through and the mozzarella has melted and is starting to turn golden. Serve with some potato wedges, cooked veg or salad.

QUICK PAN PIZZAS

Makes 4 x 20cm/8in pizzas | ❋ *Suitable for freezing (uncooked or cooked)*

These quick yeast-free pizzas are a great way to get the kids involved in the kitchen. They can be cooked on the hob or in the oven. The dough will keep in the fridge for up to three days or can be frozen in portioned balls.

350g/12oz self-raising flour, plus extra for dusting

½ tsp bicarbonate of soda

¾ tsp sea salt

350g/12oz plain full-fat live yoghurt

1 tbsp olive oil, plus extra for frying and drizzling

For the tomato sauce

200ml/7fl oz passata

1 tbsp tomato purée

1 tbsp olive oil

1 tsp dried oregano

1. To make the pizza dough, mix together the flour, bicarbonate of soda and salt in a large bowl. Make a well in the centre and mix in the yoghurt and olive oil, first with a fork and then your hands, to make a dough. Tip the dough out on to a lightly floured worktop and knead for 5 minutes into a smooth ball.

2. Put the dough back in the cleaned bowl, cover with cling film and leave to rest for 20 minutes. While the dough is resting, mix together all the ingredients for the tomato sauce and set aside.

3. Preheat the grill to high. Divide the dough into four and roll each quarter into a ball. Take one piece of dough and roll it out on a lightly floured surface to a thin round about 20cm/8in wide.

4. To cook on the hob, wipe some olive oil over the base of a large ovenproof frying pan and warm over a medium heat. When the oil is hot, place a pizza base in the pan and press it out to the edge with your fingers, taking care not to burn yourself. Cook for 2 minutes or until the base is light golden underneath. Smear a quarter of the tomato sauce over and scatter with your toppings (see opposite).

5. Drizzle a little olive oil over the top and place the pan under the grill for 5 minutes until the topping is cooked. Repeat for the remaining pizzas.

6. If baking the pizzas, preheat the oven to 220°C/425°F/ Gas 7. Roll out the dough and top with the tomato sauce and toppings. Place on a heated baking sheet and cook, two at a time, for 10–12 minutes or until the base is golden and crisp and the topping is bubbling and browning at the edges.

Topping ideas

* Thinly sliced mushrooms, red onion rings, olives and mozzarella
* Roasted peppers from a jar, cooked chicken and mozzarella
* Spinach, garlic, cream cheese and egg
* Pesto, cherry tomatoes, mozzarella and pine nuts
* Rocket, cherry tomatoes, olives and mozzarella
* Refried beans, roasted vegetables and feta
* Ricotta, peach and honey
* Blueberry, cream cheese and honey

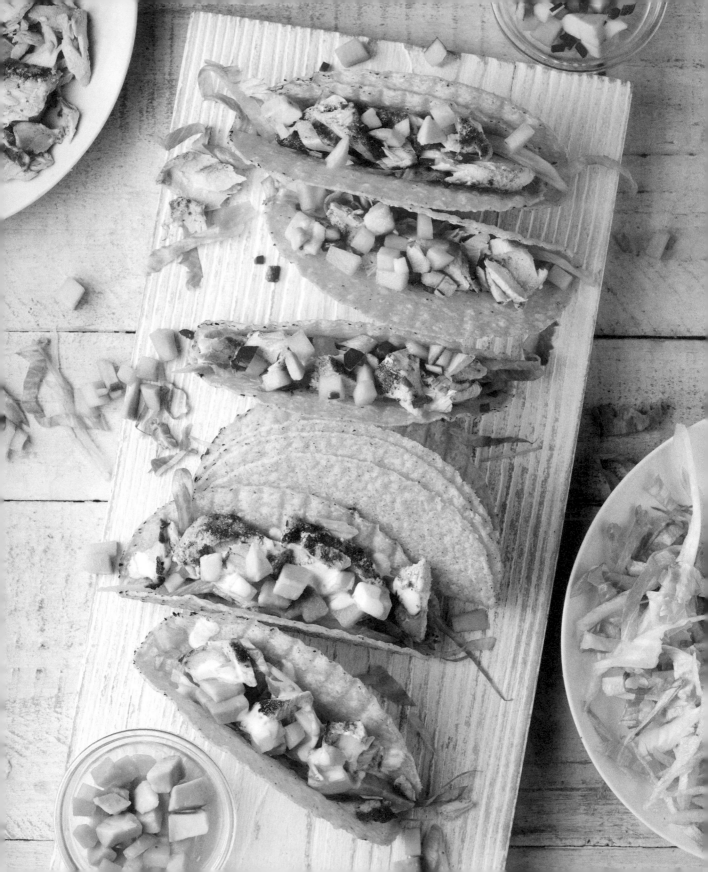

FRIDAY-NIGHT SALMON TACOS

Serves 4 (2 young children + 2 adults)

A perfect end-of-the week dinner when you don't feel like spending lots of time in the kitchen. All the various bits and pieces can be placed in separate dishes on the table for everyone to help themselves and build their own tacos.

1 tbsp olive oil

4 skinless, boneless salmon
  fillets

For the spice mix

1 tsp ground cumin

1 tsp dried oregano

2 tsp paprika

1 tsp garlic powder

For the mango and avocado salsa

Flesh of 1 small ripe mango,
  diced

Flesh of 1 small ripe avocado,
  diced

Juice of ½–1 lime

½ red onion, diced

1 fresh red chilli, deseeded and
  diced (for adults – optional)

2 tbsp finely chopped fresh
  coriander leaves

To serve

Corn taco shells or soft corn
  tortillas

Shredded crisp lettuce

Full-fat soured cream

1. Preheat the grill to medium-high and line a large baking tray with foil.
2. To make the salsa, mix together the mango and avocado, adding enough lime juice to taste. Save the red onion, chilli and coriander leaves to mix in to the grown-up portion, if you prefer.
3. Mix together the oil and the spice mix ingredients in a large shallow bowl. Add the salmon and turn in the spiced oil (you can leave out the spices for your baby's portion). Put the fish on a baking tray and grill for 8–10 minutes, turning halfway through, until the salmon is cooked. Set aside, covered with foil, to keep warm.
4. To assemble the tacos, first warm the taco shells or corn tortillas in the oven following the packet instructions. Put some shredded lettuce into each taco. Flake the salmon and add to the tacos, then top with some of the salsa and a dollop of soured cream.

227

» Salmon is rich in vitamins B and D, as well as heart-friendly omega-3 fatty acids.

CRISPY CRUMB AND PRAWN SPAGHETTI

Serves 4 (2 young children + 2 adults)

A perfect light and summery pasta dish that takes just minutes to make. If courgettes aren't a favourite, you could swap them for fine green beans, sugar snap peas or small broccoli florets. Likewise, you could use strips of cooked chicken instead of the prawns. Sprinkle the crispy crumb topping over just before serving so it keeps its crunch.

325g/11½oz dried spaghetti

125g/4½oz frozen peas

1 tbsp olive oil

2 courgettes, grated

250g/9oz cooked, peeled large prawns

1 large garlic clove, finely chopped

Juice of 1 lemon

For the crispy crumb topping

1 thick slice of day-old wholemeal bread, crusts removed, torn into pieces

1 tbsp olive oil

1 garlic clove, finely chopped

Finely grated zest of ½ unwaxed lemon

To serve (for the grown-ups – optional)

Dried chilli flakes, for sprinkling

2 handfuls of rocket leaves

1. Cook the spaghetti in plenty of unsalted boiling water following the packet instructions. Add the peas 3 minutes before the end of the cooking time and return the water to the boil. Drain over a bowl, saving 100ml/3½fl oz of the cooking water.

2. Meanwhile, make the crispy crumb topping. Blitz the bread into coarse breadcrumbs in a food processor. Heat the oil in a large frying pan, add the breadcrumbs and fry over a medium heat for 3 minutes, stirring constantly so they don't burn. Reduce the heat slightly, add the garlic and lemon zest, and cook for another minute. Tip the garlicky crumbs into a bowl and set aside to cool, then wipe the pan clean.

3. Heat the olive oil in the cleaned frying pan, add the courgettes, prawns and garlic, and cook over a medium heat for 1 minute. Add the lemon juice, along with the saved cooking water, spaghetti and peas, then turn everything with kitchen tongs or a pair of forks until mixed together.

4. Serve the prawn spaghetti sprinkled with the garlicky crumbs. Grown-ups may like to add a sprinkling of chilli flakes and a handful of rocket leaves.

CHICKEN STICKS WITH SATAY DIP

Serves 3 (young children) | ✻ *Suitable for freezing (satay dip only)*

A real winner with kids and so easy to make, these golden polenta-coated chicken sticks come with a quick satay dip. To turn this into a more substantial meal, you could serve the chicken with a vegetable noodle stir-fry, adding the satay dip to make a sauce.

Olive oil, for greasing

1 egg

75g/3oz fine polenta

225g/8oz skinless, boneless chicken thighs, cut into 1cm/½in-wide strips

Cucumber and red pepper sticks, to serve

For the satay dip

4 tbsp smooth peanut butter

1 garlic clove, crushed

1 tsp low-salt soy sauce

100ml/3½fl oz coconut drinking milk (from a carton)

Large pinch of dried chilli flakes (for the grown-ups – optional)

1. Preheat the oven to 200°C/400°F/Gas 6 and generously grease a large baking tray with olive oil.
2. Lightly beat the egg in a shallow dish and pour the polenta into a separate bowl.
3. Dip the chicken pieces into the egg, one at a time, then dunk in the polenta until coated all over. Place the chicken on the baking tray, spreading it out evenly. Bake in the oven for 20 minutes, turning halfway, until crisp and golden.
4. While the chicken is cooking, make the satay dip. Put all the ingredients in a small pan and heat gently, stirring, until warmed through and the sauce has thickened. (Grown-ups may like to add the chilli flakes to their portion at this stage.) Divide among ramekins or small bowls and serve with the chicken and the cucumber and red pepper sticks for dunking.

WEEKDAY CHICKEN ROAST

Serves 4 (2 young children + 2 adults)

This simple roast takes very little preparation – you pretty much bung the chicken thighs in the oven with the new potatoes, onion wedges and cherry tomatoes, and let it do its thing. The potatoes are in their skins, so no time-consuming peeling and you also retain more fibre. The roast comes with a moreish garlicky yoghurt sauce instead of gravy and goes really well with some fresh green veggies.

550g/1lb 4oz baby new potatoes (unpeeled)

1 large onion, peeled and cut into thick wedges with the root end still attached

1 tbsp olive oil

1 tsp dried thyme

20g/¾oz unsalted butter, softened

6 chicken thighs on the bone (skin on)

3 garlic cloves (unpeeled)

12 cherry tomatoes

Juice of 1 lemon, plus extra if needed

4 tbsp thick plain full-fat live yoghurt

1 tbsp mayonnaise

1. Preheat the oven to 200°C/400°F/Gas 6.
2. Put the potatoes and onion in a large bowl with the olive oil and toss until coated. Tip into a large roasting tin (you may need to use two tins as you want everything spread out so the skin on the potatoes and chicken crisp up).
3. Mix the thyme into the butter and dot over the top of each chicken thigh. Place the thighs in the roasting tin with the potatoes, onion and garlic cloves, and roast for 20 minutes. Remove the tin from the oven and take out the garlic if tender. Place the tomatoes around the potatoes and squeeze over the lemon juice.
4. Return the tin to the oven to roast for another 25 minutes or until the chicken is cooked through and the potatoes are tender and crisp.
5. Meanwhile, squeeze the garlic cloves out of their papery skin and mash with the back of a fork. Stir the garlic into the yoghurt and mayonnaise, adding a splash of water or lemon juice to loosen. Serve the chicken roast with a spoonful of the yoghurt sauce by the side.

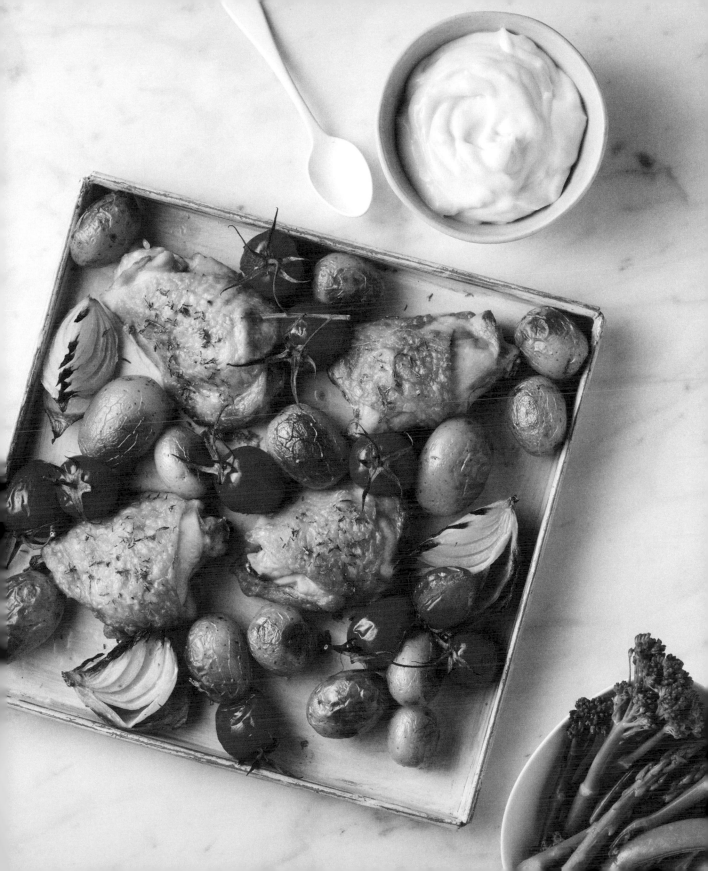

LAMB AND BULGUR WHEAT PILAF

Serves 4–6 (2–3 young children + 2–3 adults) | ❋ *Suitable for freezing*

I've added cooked lamb to this tomatoey bulgur pilaf, but any leftover roast meat, such as chicken, beef or pork, would work well. And, if you want to serve it as a veggie meal, top it with a poached egg, or cubes of smoke tofu or a handful of toasted chopped almonds. A spoonful of the mint yoghurt on top adds the finishing touch.

1 tbsp olive oil

1 large onion, finely chopped

2 garlic cloves, finely chopped

50g/2oz cauliflower florets, grated

175g/6oz bulgur wheat

1 tbsp tomato purée

400g/14oz tin of chopped tomatoes

300ml/11fl oz low-salt chicken stock (for homemade Bone Broth, see page 111)

250g/9oz leftover roast lamb, chopped

1 handful of chopped fresh parsley leaves

Dried chilli flakes, for sprinkling (for the grown-ups – optional)

For the mint yoghurt

6 tbsp thick plain full-fat live yoghurt

3 tbsp finely chopped fresh mint leaves

Juice of ½ lemon

1 small garlic clove, finely chopped

1. Heat the olive oil in a saucepan, add the onion and stir-fry over a medium heat for 8 minutes or until softened. Turn the heat down slightly, stir in the garlic and cauliflower, and cook for another minute.
2. Stir in the bulgur wheat, tomato purée, chopped tomatoes and stock. Bring almost to bubbling point, then reduce the heat to low, cover the pan and simmer for 20 minutes or until the bulgur wheat is tender and all the liquid has been absorbed. Stir in the cooked lamb and parsley, cover again with the lid and leave to sit for 5 minutes.
3. While the pilaf is cooking, mix together all the ingredients for the mint yoghurt. Serve the pilaf topped with a spoonful of the mint yoghurt. Grown-ups may like to add a sprinkling of dried chilli flakes.

THAI PORK STIR-FRY

Serves 4 (2 young children + 2 adults) | ❄ *Suitable for freezing*

This stir-fry captures the flavours of Thai cooking but without being overly spicy and hot. Don't be put off by the long list of ingredients – it's really very easy and, being a complete meal, you don't need anything else to go with it.

1 onion, roughly chopped

2 garlic cloves (peeled)

2.5cm/1in piece of fresh root ginger, roughly chopped (no need to peel)

1 lemongrass stick (outer layer removed), roughly chopped

Juice of 1 lime

1 tbsp low-salt soy sauce

1 tsp honey

1 tbsp coconut or groundnut oil

300g/11oz lean pork mince

2 kaffir lime leaves (optional)

1 small red pepper, deseeded and chopped

75g/3oz sugar snap peas

60g/2½oz baby corn, cut in half lengthways

200g/7oz medium egg noodles

To serve (optional)

1 fresh red chilli, deseeded and thinly sliced (for the grown-ups)

40g/1½oz roasted peanuts, finely chopped

1. Put the onion, garlic, ginger and lemongrass in a food processor or blender and blend to a paste before setting aside. Mix together the lime juice, soy sauce and honey in a small bowl and set aside.

2. Heat the coconut or groundnut oil in a wok or large frying pan, add the mince and stir-fry over a high heat for 5 minutes or until browned. Add the kaffir lime leaves (if using) and the onion paste, and cook, stirring, for another 3 minutes. Toss in the red pepper, sugar snaps and baby corn, and stir-fry for a further 3–5 minutes or until softened.

3. Meanwhile, cook the noodles in plenty of unsalted boiling water following the packet instructions, then drain over a bowl, saving 100ml/3½fl oz of the cooking water. Add the noodles to the wok or frying pan, along with the saved cooking water and soy sauce mixture, and toss until combined and warmed through. Serve sprinkled with the chopped peanuts and chilli, if you like.

COCONUT AND PASSION FRUIT FRO-YOS

Makes about 8 (depending on the size of the lolly moulds)

Made with fresh passion fruit, lime juice, apple and coconut, these lollies are both healthy – passion fruit is high in vitamin C – and full of zingy flavour. I've left the passion fruit seeds in, but you could press the fruit pulp through a sieve if you prefer a smoother fruit purée.

3 passion fruit, halved

1 tbsp maple syrup

4 tbsp fresh apple juice (not from concentrate)

Squeeze of lime juice

125g/4½oz thick plain coconut yoghurt or tinned coconut milk

You will need about 8 ice-lolly moulds and lolly sticks

1. Using a teaspoon, scoop out the passion fruit pulp into a bowl, then stir in the maple syrup, apple juice and lime juice.
2. Pour half of the passion fruit mixture into your ice-lolly moulds, top with the coconut yoghurt or coconut milk and then pour in the rest of the passion fruit mixture, filling each mould almost to the top.
3. Pop in the lolly sticks and freeze for about 5 hours or until firm. Remove from the freezer about 10 minutes before you want to serve the lollies, so they have time to soften slightly.

MANGO SOUP WITH FRUIT BAUBLES

Serves 4 (2 young children + 2 adults)

No one will know that this sweet fruit soup contains beetroot if you don't tell them, but it does give the pudding a wonderful colour . . .

2 bananas, peeled and sliced

1 large ripe mango

1 cooked beetroot (not in vinegar; about 60g/2½oz)

1 handful of blueberries

1. Put the bananas in a freezer-proof container and freeze for about 3 hours or until firm but not completely frozen.
2. Cut the mango away from the central stone and reserve a quarter. Scoop out or cut away the mango flesh from the skin, and put it in a blender with the beetroot and frozen bananas. Blend until smooth and pour into four small bowls.
3. Cut the reserved mango into small pieces (or scoop into balls using a small melon baller) and scatter over the top with the blueberries. Serve chilled.

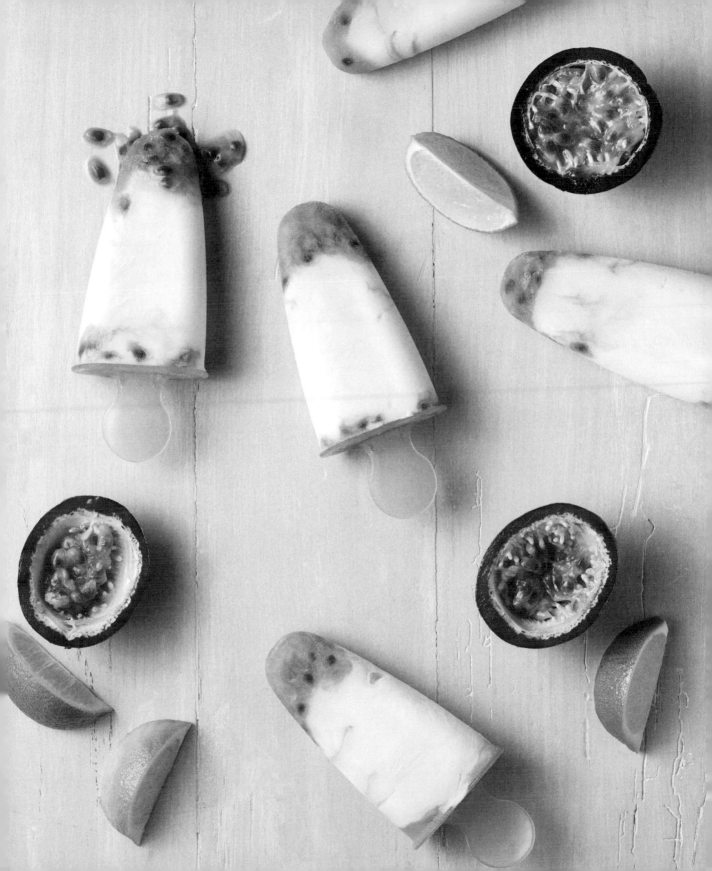

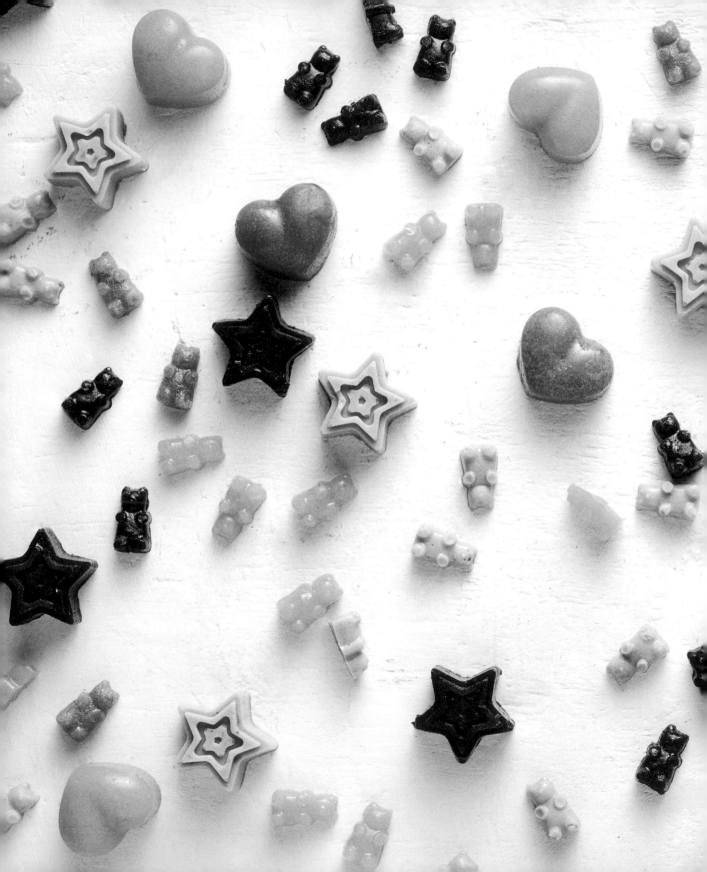

STRAWBERRY GUMMY BEARS

Makes about 18 sweets (depending on the size of the mould)

Check the ingredients list on most packets of jelly sweets and it's an alarming mix of sugar and artificial colourings and flavourings. Made with fresh strawberries, these natural alternatives are no less delicious but with the added bonus of being completely additive-free. They're bear-shaped but if you don't have a bear mould (find online), select your child's favourite shape or whatever is convenient – you could even use an ice-cube tray or chocolate mould.

I've given other flavour options using different blends of fruit and veg (see the variations on page 238), but all are made in pretty much the same way and contain a little honey for sweetness as well as powdered gelatine as a setting agent. Be aware that since fruit and honey contain natural sugars, the gummies are still treats.

160g/5½oz strawberries, hulled and chopped

½ tsp lemon juice

2 tbsp honey

3 tsp powdered gelatine

You will need a bear-shaped mould or other shape of baking mould, or an ice-cube tray

1. Put the strawberries in a blender, or use a hand blender, and purée until smooth. Pour the purée into a small saucepan, add the lemon juice and honey, and heat gently until hot but not boiling. Remove from the heat and gradually stir in the gelatine, stirring well with a wooden spoon. If the gelatine doesn't dissolve fully, return the pan briefly to the heat but don't let the purée boil.
2. Place the bear moulds, or your chosen shape of mould, on a baking tray, pour in the strawberry jelly and chill in the fridge for a few hours or until set. Pop the gummy bears out of the moulds and store in a lidded container in the fridge for up to one week.

* Mango and carrot: Make as on page 237, swapping the strawberries for 1 small chopped carrot and 100g/3½oz mango flesh and adding 1–2 tablespoons of honey to taste.

* Black grape and beetroot: Make as on page 237, replacing the strawberries with 100g/3½oz seedless black grapes and 50g/2oz chopped cooked beetroot (not in vinegar) and adding 1–2 tablespoons of honey to taste.

* Raspberry cream: Swap the strawberries for 100g/3½oz raspberries and make as on page 237. Allow the purée to cool slightly and stir in 2 tablespoons of thick plain full-fat live yoghurt before pouring into the moulds.

CHOCOLATE PUDDLES WITH FRUIT KEBABS

Serves 4 (2 young children + 2 adults)

These little pots of chocolate heaven – made with no added sugar – are perfect for dunking the fruit kebabs into. The fruit is threaded on to cocktail sticks, though for young children it's best to leave these out. Instead arrange a selection of 'dunkable' fruit on a plate and let them help themselves. Messy, but par for the course!

For the chocolate puddles

2 ripe bananas, peeled and sliced

4 soft pitted dates, roughly chopped

Flesh of 1 small ripe avocado

100ml/3½fl oz full-fat milk

2 tsp vanilla extract

2 tbsp cocoa or cacao powder

For the fruit kebabs

Selection of fresh fruit (such as strawberries, clementine segments, kiwi slices, seedless grapes, or chunks of mango, apple or pear)

You will need cocktail sticks or small wooden skewers

1. First make the chocolate puddles. Put the bananas in a freezer-proof container and freeze for about 3 hours or until firm but not completely frozen.
2. Put the dates in a small bowl, pour enough hot water over to cover and leave to soak for 2 hours.
3. Drain the dates and put them in a blender (or use a hand blender) with the frozen bananas and remaining ingredients and blend until smooth and creamy. Spoon the chocolate mixture into four large ramekins or similar-sized bowls and chill in the fridge for 30 minutes or until ready to serve.
4. To make the fruit kebabs, thread a selection of fresh fruit pieces on to cocktail sticks or small wooden skewers (leave out the sticks/skewers for young children). Have fun dunking them into the chocolate puddles.

RASPBERRY BABY CHEESECAKES

Makes about 8 cheesecakes | ❋ Suitable for freezing (without the raspberry topping)

These are just the perfect size for young children and are conveniently made in a deep muffin tin. They come with a scattering of fresh raspberries but feel free to swap for your own favourite fruit – mango, strawberries, peaches and nectarines would all taste delicious. Just bear in mind that they should be regarded as a treat and, because of the sugar and salt in the digestive biscuits, not given to children under one year of age.

40g/1½oz butter, plus extra for greasing

60g/2½oz digestive biscuits

20g/¾oz pecan nuts

200g/7oz fresh raspberries

1 tbsp maple syrup

For the filling

175g/6oz full-fat cream cheese

75g/3oz thick plain full-fat live yoghurt

Finely grated zest of 1 unwaxed lemon and 2 tbsp juice

2 tbsp maple syrup

2 tsp vanilla extract

1 egg, lightly beaten

1 tsp cornflour

You will need a deep 12-hole muffin tin

1. Preheat the oven to 160°C/315°F/Gas 2½ and grease 8 holes of the muffin tin with butter. To make the cheesecakes easier to lift out of the tin, cut 16 long strips of baking paper, about 13cm/5in wide, and fold in half lengthways. Place two strips crossways in each muffin hole, so they rise above the hole and can be used as 'handles'.

2. To make the base, put the digestives and pecans in a food processor and blitz to coarse crumbs. Gently melt the butter in a small saucepan and then stir it into the biscuit and pecan mixture. Divide the mixture evenly among the prepared holes of the muffin tin and press down with the back of a teaspoon to make a firm, even base. Bake in the oven for 10 minutes until just crisp.

3. Meanwhile, beat together all the ingredients for the filling until smooth and creamy. Pour the filling into the muffin tin over the biscuit base, leaving a small amount of space on top. Place in the oven to cook for 18–20 minutes or until the filling is just firm but still has a slight wobble. Leave to cool while you make the raspberry topping.

CONTINUES ON NEXT PAGE

4. Crush half of the raspberries with the back of a fork, stir in the maple syrup and then add the whole raspberries. Spoon the raspberry mixture over the cooled cheesecakes, so it fills each mould to the top, and then chill in the fridge for at least 30 minutes.
5. When you are ready to serve, lift out the cheesecakes, using the strips of baking paper to help you, and place on individual plates.

EASIEST BANANA PUDDING EVER

Serves 2 (young children)

If you're looking for a speedy pudding, then this is for you. Cinnamon is a brilliant way of adding natural sweetness, eliminating the need for lots of added sugar.

2 tsp coconut oil or butter

2 small ripe bananas, peeled and sliced in half lengthways

1 tsp maple syrup or honey (optional)

¼ tsp ground cinnamon (optional)

Thick plain full-fat live yoghurt, to serve

1. Melt the coconut oil or butter in a small frying pan. Add the bananas and spoon over the melted oil or butter. Cook over a medium heat for 3 minutes, turning once, until softened.
2. Transfer the bananas to serving plates. Turn the heat down to low and add the maple syrup or honey and cinnamon (if using) to the pan. Heat through briefly, stirring, then spoon the mixture over the bananas. Serve with a good spoonful of yoghurt.

» Bananas contain tryptophan, a relaxant that aids sleep, and, like live yoghurt, they benefit the digestive system.

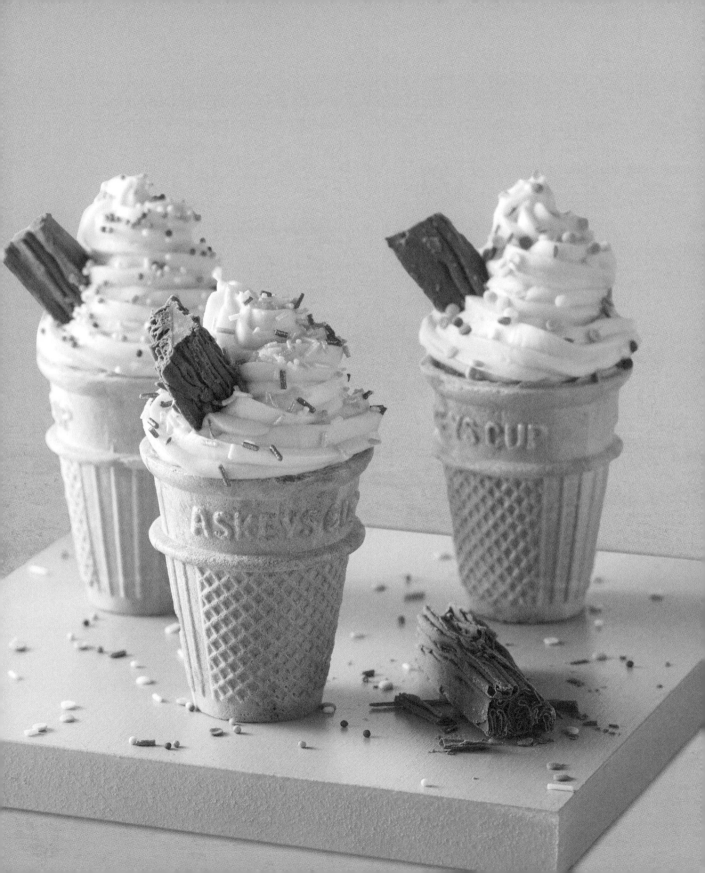

Chapter 7

PARTY TIME

Celebrations call for a little indulgence, as we all know. In this chapter, I've provided some of my favourite recipes for birthdays and get-togethers, and some of them are a little higher in sugar than you would tend to feed your little ones day to day. Ice-cream Cone Cakes (see page 259) and the Garden Birthday Cake (see page 256) are particularly indulgent, so try to stick to moderate portions!

That said, I don't think you can go through life without having treats now and again – in fact, those experiences are just as valid a part of childhood as healthy dining. If you severely limit or ban certain things completely, your child might start to gravitate towards them when they're old enough to make their own choices, and they might do so to excess.

There are plenty of healthy options here, too, though. I've included a few fun ideas about how to use the shape and colour of fresh fruit and veg to make plates of party canapés that are as tasty as they are eye-catching. Sweet cherry tomatoes can be transformed into ladybirds (see page 249), cucumbers turned into castles (see page 252) and wedges of apple into scary monster mouths (see page 246)!

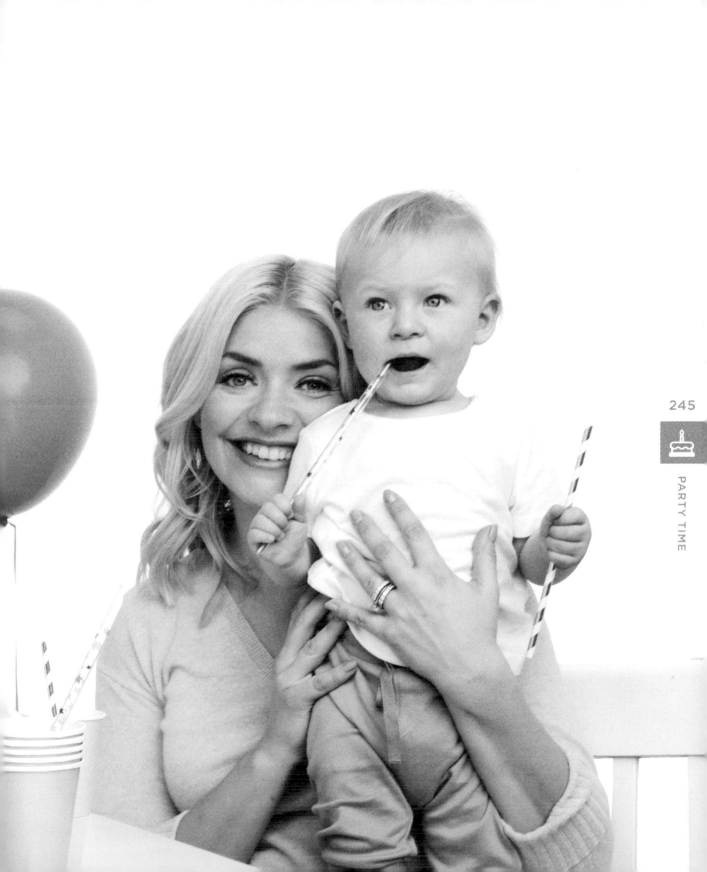

APPLE MONSTER MOUTHS

Makes 8 'mouths'

Great for a Halloween party and definitely one to make with the kids. These Apple Monster Mouths come with two options for the eyes: shop-bought googly eyes or homemade eye antennae made with fruit-topped cocktail sticks. It is also possible to make your own version of googly eyes using a small disc of white sugar paste (or 'ready to roll' icing) with a chocolate-chip pupil. You'll need to make these in advance to give the sugar paste time to dry.

2 green eating apples, cut into quarters and cored

Juice of 1 lemon, for brushing

3 tbsp smooth peanut butter or other nut butter (for homemade see page 280)

2 tbsp sunflower seeds (for the teeth)

2 strawberries, hulled and sliced lengthways (for the tongues)

16 ready-made googly eyes, or 16 cocktail sticks and fruit of choice for the eyes (such as seedless grapes, blueberries, big raisins/sultanas or natural-colour glacé cherries)

1. Cut a wedge lengthways out of the skin side of each apple quarter to make a mouth (with the apple skin forming green 'lips' on either side). Repeat with the rest of the apple quarters, to make eight mouths in total. Brush the cut sides of each apple wedge with lemon juice to stop them browning.

2. Spread the inside of each mouth with peanut or other nut butter and then press a few sunflower seeds into the top of the mouth to create a row of teeth. Place a slice of strawberry in the bottom of the mouth to make a tongue.

3. Using a little peanut or other nut butter, stick the googly eyes on to the top skin-side part of each apple mouth. Alternatively, place a piece of fruit on a cocktail stick and press two into the top of each mouth to make antennae eyes. Arrange the apple monsters on a serving plate.

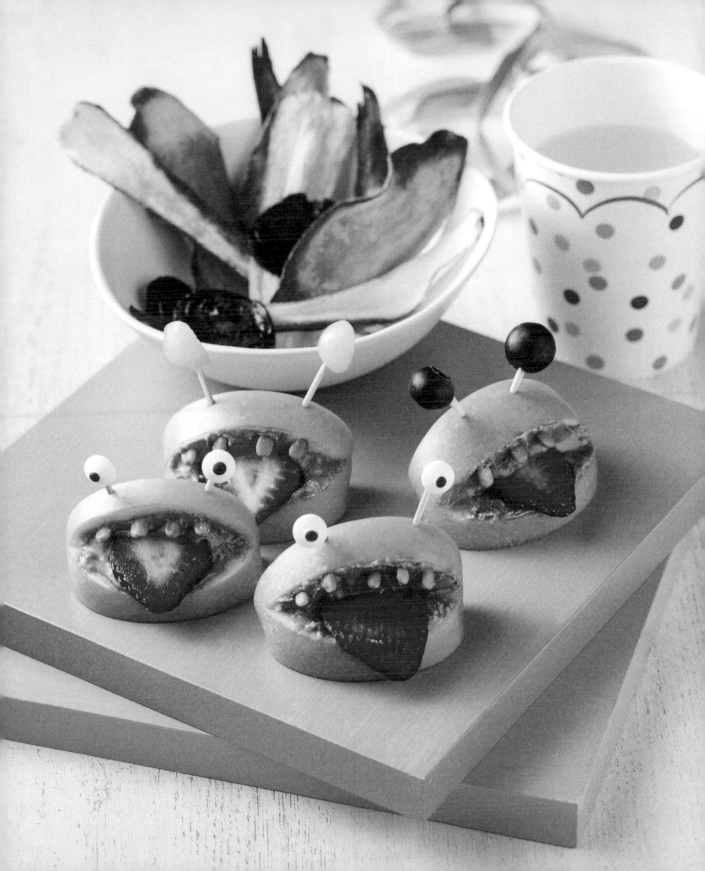

VEGETABLE RIBBONS

Serves 6–8

Colourful root veggies cut into thin ribbons and baked until crisp make a healthy alternative to regular salted potato crisps. If you have a mandolin, you can also make thin round crisps, but do watch your fingers! Feel free to experiment with other veg, too, such as carrots, celeriac or potatoes.

1 parsnip, peeled

1 small sweet potato, peeled

1 small raw beetroot, scrubbed

3 tsp sunflower oil

1. Preheat the oven to 180°C/350°F/Gas 4 and line 2–3 baking trays with baking paper.
2. Using a swivel vegetable peeler, cut the vegetables into thin, wide strips. Place between two sheets of kitchen paper and pat dry.
3. Put the vegetable ribbons in a large bowl. Put the beetroot in a separate bowl as its colour will seep into the other veg. Drizzle 1 teaspoon of the sunflower oil over the beetroot and the rest of the oil over the parsnip and sweet potato, and toss with your hands (wear gloves when touching the beetroot to avoid getting pink hands) until lightly coated all over.
4. Spread the vegetables out in a single layer on the lined baking trays (you may need to cook them in two batches) and roast in the oven for 20–30 minutes, turning once and swapping the trays around, or until crisp. Check towards the end of the cooking time, as the vegetables can burn in a blink of an eye, and remove any ribbons that are ready. Remove from the oven and place the vegetable ribbons on kitchen paper to cool and crisp up further.

Apple crisps

For a fruity alternative to the vegetable ribbons, slice 2 eating apples into 3mm/⅛in-thick rounds, brush both sides with a little sunflower oil and cook in the oven, as above, for 45 minutes, turning halfway, or until crisp.

TOMATO LADYBIRDS

Makes 10 ladybirds

These look fun at a party and are a great way to encourage children to enjoy savoury foods. You could pair these with the Garden Birthday Cake on page 256 for a complete nature-based theme.

10 baby rice cakes or oatcakes

10 small fresh basil leaves (optional)

5 small plum tomatoes, halved lengthways and the seeds scooped out

5 pitted black olives, 3 quartered crossways and the rest very finely diced

For the guacamole

Flesh of 1 small ripe avocado

1 tbsp plain full-fat live yoghurt or mayonnaise

1 small garlic clove, crushed (optional)

Juice of ½ lemon

1. Put all the ingredients for the guacamole into a bowl and use the back of a fork to mash until smooth. Place a spoonful on each rice cake or oatcake and top with a basil leaf on one side (if using).
2. To make the ladybirds, take one tomato half and lightly score the skin lengthways down the centre using the tip of a pointed knife, then cut a narrow wedge out of one end to give the appearance of two wings about to open. Sit the tomato ladybird on top of a guacamole-coated rice cake/oatcake.
3. Place an olive quarter at the top end to make a head. To make the ladybird dots, take a few of the diced olives and place them, flesh-side down, on the tomato – it's a bit of a fiddle but they should stick without extra help. Repeat to make 10 tomato ladybirds in total.

» Tomatoes are a great source of vitamin C which is important for the immune system and helps keep our teeth and skin healthy.

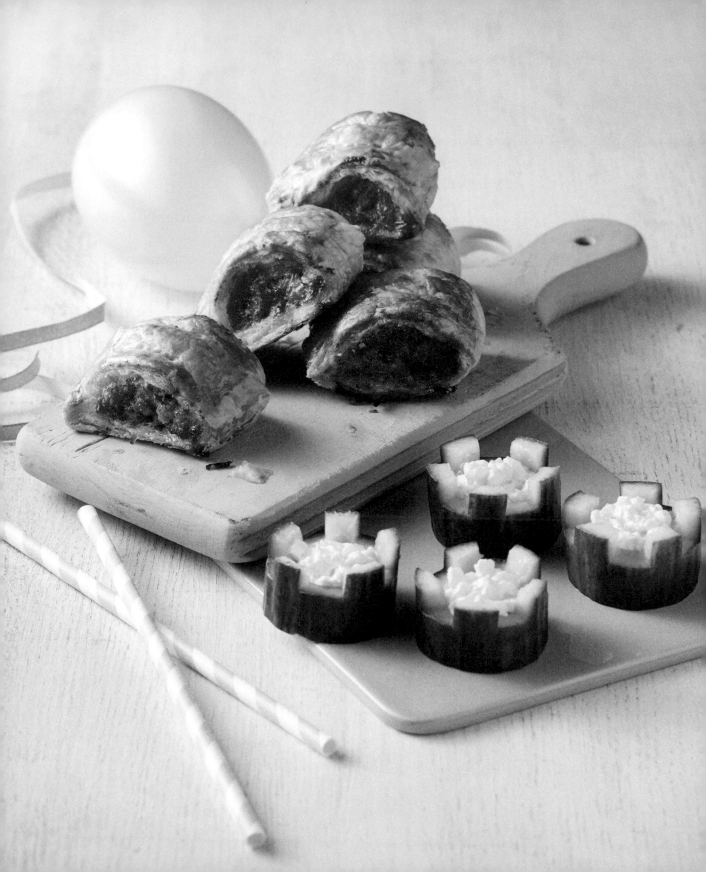

ROCKIN' ROLLS

Makes 12 sausage rolls | ✳ *Suitable for freezing (uncooked)*

You can't beat a good sausage roll and the filling for these is pimped up with carrot and ground almonds. You could make them in advance and store uncooked in the freezer – just make sure they are thoroughly defrosted before baking.

400g/14oz good-quality herby pork sausage meat

4 tbsp ground almonds

1 carrot (about 50g/2oz), scrubbed/peeled and finely grated

320g/11½oz ready-rolled puff pastry

1 egg, lightly beaten

Freshly ground black pepper

1. Preheat the oven to 200°C/400°F/Gas 6 and line a baking sheet with baking paper.
2. Mix together the sausage meat, ground almonds and carrot in a large bowl and season with pepper.
3. Unroll the pastry and cut it in half lengthways.
4. Take half of the sausage-meat mixture and spoon it lengthways down the middle of one piece of pastry in a long sausage shape, about 2cm/¾in wide. Brush one of the long edges of pastry with some of the beaten egg and then fold it over the sausage-meat filling. Press the edges together to seal and then crimp with the back of a fork.
5. Cut the filled pastry widthways into six sausage rolls, each about 5cm/2in long, and prick the tops a couple of times with a fork. Tidy up the ends of the rolls if the filling has squished out a bit and then place on the prepared baking sheet. Repeat with the remaining pastry and filling to make another six sausage rolls.
6. Brush the top of each sausage roll with the remaining beaten egg and bake in the oven for 30–35 minutes or until risen and golden. Leave to cool slightly before transferring to a wire rack. They are best eaten while still warm.

CUCUMBER CASTLES

Makes 10 castles

Scoop the seeds out of a chunk of cucumber and cut the top to make the battlements and you have a cucumber castle, just waiting to be filled with a retro mix of cream cheese and pineapple (see page 250).

25cm/10in piece of cucumber

50g/2oz full-fat cream cheese

75g/3oz fresh pineapple, core removed and flesh finely chopped

1. Cut the cucumber into ten slices, each 2.5cm/1in thick. Using a teaspoon, scoop the seeds out of each slice of cucumber, leaving the base intact, to form ten 'cups'. Using a small sharp knife, cut a crenelated top in each piece to make the battlements, so the cucumber slices look like mini castles. This is a bit fiddly but well worth it.

2. Mix together the cream cheese and pineapple, and spoon the mixture into the cucumber castles. Store in the fridge until ready to serve later in the day.

CHEESY FEET

Makes about 20 biscuits | ❊ *Suitable for freezing (uncooked or cooked)*

Fun for a party or snack, these feet-shaped savoury biscuits are flavoured with cheese! If you don't have a foot-shaped cutter, use any cutter you have to hand – even an upturned glass will work. The biscuits are made with half wholemeal and half plain flour for extra nutrients and fibre, but you could use a single type of flour, if it's easier.

75g/3oz unsalted butter, cut into small pieces, plus extra for greasing

100g/3½oz plain flour, plus extra for dusting

100g/3½oz wholemeal flour

1 tbsp ground flaxseeds/linseeds (optional)

50g/2oz ground almonds

1 tsp baking powder

75g/3oz mature Cheddar cheese, grated

1 egg, lightly beaten

4 tbsp full-fat milk, plus extra for brushing

You will need a foot-shaped pastry cutter or other shape of your choice

1. Preheat the oven to 200°C/400°F/Gas 6 and lightly grease two baking sheets with butter.
2. Put both types of flour in a large bowl with the flaxseeds, ground almonds and baking powder, and stir until combined.
3. Rub the butter in with your fingertips to make coarse crumbs, then stir in the cheese, egg and milk. Press everything together, then tip out on to a floured work surface, knead lightly and form into a ball of dough.
4. Roll out the dough to about 1cm/½in thick and, using the pastry cutter, stamp out about 20 biscuits, re-rolling the dough as needed. Place on the prepared baking sheets and brush lightly with milk. Bake in the oven for 17–20 minutes or until lightly golden and then transfer to a wire rack to cool.

FROZEN FRUITY YOGHURT CAKE

Serves 10–12

A perfect summery alternative to the usual birthday cake and it's gluten-free. The yoghurt cake is made up of layers of creamy strawberry, mango, banana and blueberry, and looks amazing, especially topped with extra fresh fruit – if you freeze them slightly before decorating, they develop a frosty bloom on the outside.

100g/3½oz plain full-fat live Greek yoghurt

150ml/5fl oz double cream

4 tsp vanilla extract

250g/9oz ripe strawberries, hulled

3 tbsp honey

250g/9oz blueberries

2 large ripe bananas, peeled and cut into chunks

Flesh of 1 large ripe mango, chopped

You will need a 900g/2lb loaf tin

1. Line the loaf tin with cling film, leaving enough hanging over the edges to cover the top of the tin. Try to smooth out as many creases as you can.
2. Mix together the yoghurt, cream and vanilla extract in a bowl.
3. Set aside 50g/2oz of the strawberries to decorate the top of the cake and blitz the rest in a blender with 4 tablespoons of the yoghurt mixture and 1 tablespoon of the honey. Spoon the mixture into the lined loaf tin and freeze for 30 minutes or until it starts to set.
4. Set aside 50g/2oz of the blueberries to decorate the top of the cake and blend the rest with 4 tablespoons of the yoghurt mixture and 1 tablespoon of the honey. Spoon the mixture into the loaf tin on top of the strawberry layer and freeze for 30 minutes or until it starts to set.
5. Blend the bananas with 4 tablespoons of the yoghurt mixture – you don't need to add any honey as they will be sweet enough. Spoon the mixture on top of the blueberry layer and freeze for 30 minutes or until starting to set.

CONTINUES ON NEXT PAGE

6. Set aside a quarter of the mango to decorate the top of the cake and blend the rest with the remaining yoghurt mixture and honey. Spoon the mixture on top of the banana layer, cover the top with the overhanging cling film and freeze until firm.

7. Remove the yoghurt cake from the freezer 20–30 minutes before serving to let it soften slightly. Lift it out of the loaf tin, using the overhanging cling film to help, and invert on a serving plate. Peel off the cling film and decorate the top with the saved strawberries, blueberries and mango. Serve cut into slices.

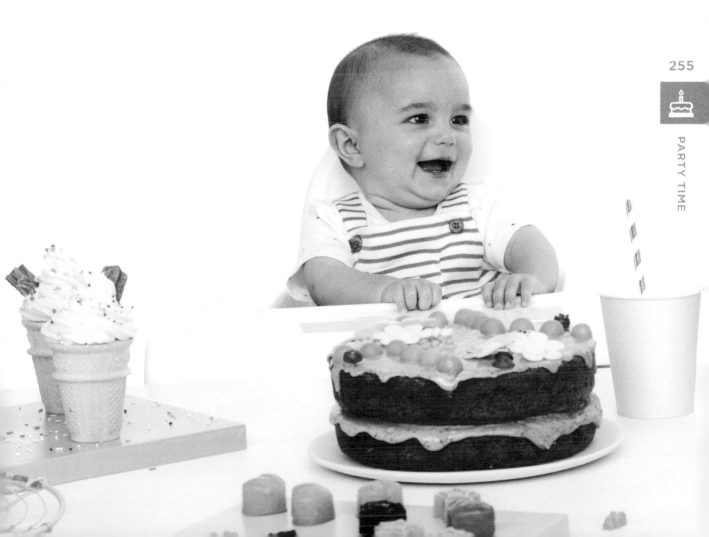

GARDEN BIRTHDAY CAKE

Serves about 12 | ❄ *Suitable for freezing (unfrosted)*

Vegetables not only add valuable vitamins and minerals to this stunning cake but they keep it lovely and moist, too. The double-layered cake – carrot and beetroot – is topped with a pink cream-cheese frosting, coloured with beetroot (if you want a plain vanilla icing, just leave out the beetroot). Stick to the garden theme and decorate the cake with edible flowers, a caterpillar made with green grapes, or other nature-related treats.

250g/9oz self-raising flour

1 tsp baking powder

1 tsp mixed spice

225g/8oz unrefined light brown soft sugar

4 eggs

200ml/7fl oz sunflower oil

Finely grated zest of 1 unwaxed orange

125g/4½oz carrot, scrubbed and coarsely grated

125g/4½oz raw beetroot, scrubbed and coarsely grated

For the icing

100g/3½oz unsalted butter, softened, plus extra for greasing

200g/7oz full-fat cream cheese

1 tsp vanilla extract

100g/3½oz unrefined light brown soft sugar

40g/1½oz raw beetroot, scrubbed and finely grated and excess liquid squeezed out (optional)

1. Preheat the oven to 180°C/350°F/Gas 4, then lightly grease the sides of each cake tin and line each base with a disc of baking paper.
2. Sift the flour, baking powder and mixed spice into a large bowl and add the sugar. Stir until combined and make a well in the centre.
3. Whisk together the eggs, sunflower oil and orange zest, then stir it into the flour mixture using a wooden spoon. Divide the mixture between two bowls and stir the grated carrot into one bowl and the grated beetroot into the other.
4. Pour the carrot-cake mixture into one of the prepared tins and the beetroot-cake mixture into the other. Bake in the oven for 30–40 minutes or until a skewer inserted into the centre of each cake comes out clean. Remove from the oven and allow to cool for 10 minutes before removing from the tins and transferring to a wire rack to cool down fully.
5. While the cakes are baking, make the icing. Using an electric whisk, beat together the butter and vanilla extract until smooth and creamy. Beat in the sugar until combined then fold in the cream cheese and the beetroot (if using), to colour it pink (or leave plain, if you prefer). Chill in the fridge to firm up.

CONTINUES ON NEXT PAGE

For the decoration

About 10 seedless green grapes,
and a tube of black writing
icing (for the caterpillar)

Edible organic flowers

Other edible garden-themed
decorations

*You will need two 20cm/8in round
spring-form cake tins*

6. To decorate the cake, place the beetroot cake on a
serving plate or cake stand and spread over half of
the frosting. Top with the carrot cake and spread the
remaining frosting over the top. You can pop it in the
fridge at this point (it will keep in the fridge for up to a
day) or finish decorating, if serving within a few hours.

7. To make a grape caterpillar, cut the grapes in half and
arrange in a curvy line on the top of the cake. Using
a tube of black writing icing, make two blobs for eyes.
Decorate with edible flowers and/or other garden-
themed decorations.

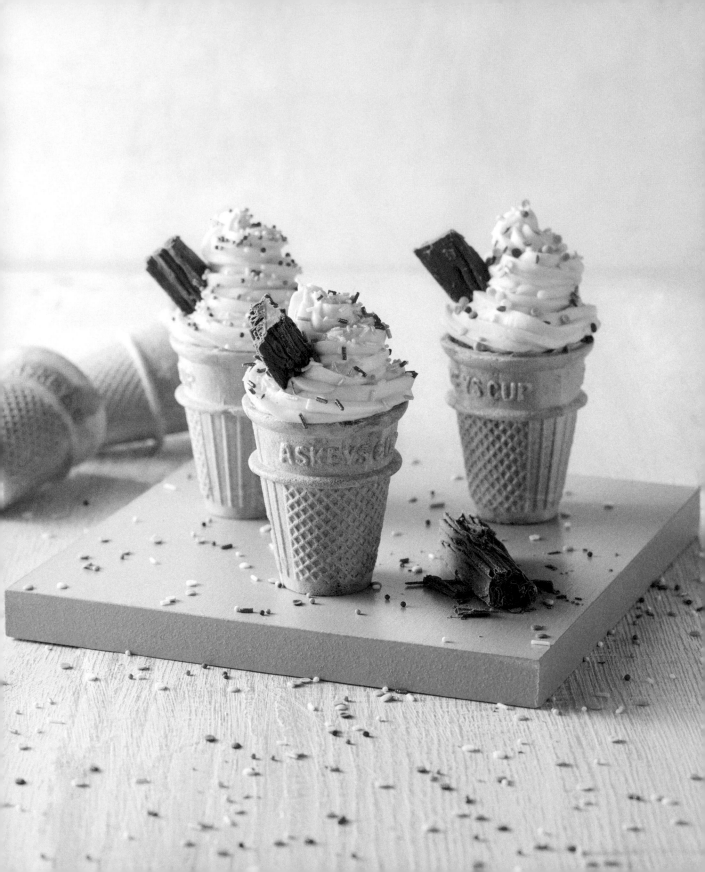

ICE-CREAM CONE CAKES

Makes 10–12 cakes

An ice-cream cone, rather than the usual paper one, makes a surprisingly good case for a light vanilla muffin. Each cone is topped with whipped buttercream icing and sprinkles – you could even add a flake!

10–12 flat-bottomed ice-cream cones (depending on size)

175g/6oz butter, softened

175g/6oz caster sugar

1 tsp vanilla extract

3 eggs

175g/6oz self-raising flour

50g/2oz ground almonds

Sprinkles, edible glitter and chocolate flakes, to decorate

For the buttercream icing

300g/11oz butter, softened

300g/11oz icing sugar, sifted

2 tsp vanilla extract

You will need a deep 12-hole muffin tin and a piping bag with a large plain nozzle and a large star nozzle

1. Preheat the oven to 180°C/350°F/Gas 4 and place the ice-cream cones in the holes of the muffin tin. Add scrunched-up pieces of baking paper around the base of each cone to help to keep them steady.
2. Using an electric whisk, beat the butter and sugar until pale and creamy. Beat in the vanilla extract and the eggs, one at a time, scraping the bowl down after each addition and adding a spoonful of the flour if the mixture starts to split.
3. Using a metal spoon, fold in the flour and the ground almonds in two batches to make a smooth cake batter. Spoon or pipe the mixture into the ice-cream cones (it may help to ask someone to hold the cones for you) until three-quarters full and make sure the batter reaches the bottom of the cone. Bake in the oven for 30–35 minutes or until risen and golden and a skewer inserted into the middle comes out clean.
4. Using an electric whisk or a food processor, whisk all the buttercream ingredients together for 3–4 minutes until smooth and fluffy. Spoon the buttercream into a piping bag fitted with a large star nozzle. Using a spiral motion, pipe the buttercream on the top of each ice-cream cake in a large swirl. Decorate with your choice of sprinkles and edible glitter and add a chocolate flake.

GIANT CHOCOLATE BUTTONS

Makes 10 sweets

Use your imagination when decorating these chocolate treats and get the kids to help out, too. You can go down the healthy route with freeze-dried fruit or chopped nuts, or go glitzy with colourful sprinkles and edible glitter. You could also swirl together melted milk, plain and white chocolate to get a lovely marbled effect.

150g/5oz good-quality milk chocolate, broken into even-sized chunks

Topping ideas

Freeze-dried raspberries or strawberries

Chopped dried fruit

Toasted seeds or chopped toasted nuts

Sprinkles or edible glitter

1. Line two large baking sheets with baking paper and draw ten circles on the paper using a 5cm/2in-diameter glass or pastry cutter as a guide. Turn the paper over.
2. To melt the chocolate, place it in a heatproof bowl set over a saucepan of gently simmering water. (Do not let the bottom of the bowl touch the water or allow the water to boil.) Stir once or twice until the chocolate melts, then carefully lift the bowl out of the pan. Leave to cool for a couple of minutes.
3. To make the buttons, place a large spoonful of the melted chocolate in the middle of one of the circles on the baking paper, then spread it out with a palette knife or paint brush. Repeat to make ten buttons in total.
4. Sprinkle the top of the buttons with your choice of decoration, then leave to cool and set (you can put them in the fridge if the weather is warm). Once firm, peel the chocolate buttons off the paper.

Chocolate lollipops

You can also make chocolate lollipops using this recipe. Simply lay a lolly stick in each circle of melted chocolate, so that half of the stick is pressed into the chocolate and the other half is sticking out, then decorate as you like and leave until firm.

MINI CHOCOLATE-CHERRY MUFFINS

Makes 12 mini muffins | ❋ *Suitable for freezing*

These gluten-free muffins are super-simple to make and you can't beat the combination of chocolate and cherries.

4 tbsp sunflower oil

3 eggs, lightly beaten

1 tsp vanilla extract

4 tbsp maple syrup

100g/3½oz ground almonds

1 heaped tsp baking powder (gluten-free, if you prefer)

25g/1oz cocoa or cacao powder

40g/1½oz dried cherries, finely chopped

You will need a 12-hole mini muffin tin and paper cases

1. Preheat the oven to 180°C/350°F/Gas 4 and line the muffin tin with paper cases.
2. Place the sunflower oil in a jug with the eggs, vanilla extract and maple syrup, and whisk together.
3. Mix together the ground almonds, baking powder, cocoa/cacao powder and cherries in a large bowl. Make a well in the centre and gently fold in the sunflower oil and egg mixture to make a cake batter.
4. Spoon the batter into the paper cases and bake in the oven for 15–20 minutes or until well risen and firm to the touch. Transfer to a wire rack to cool.

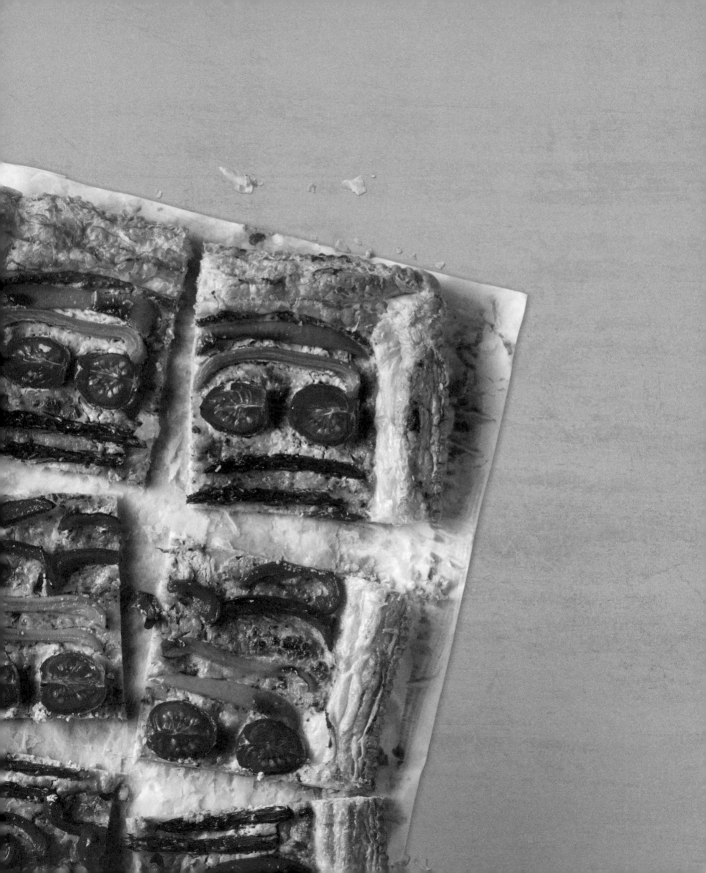

Chapter 8

FEEDING THE WHOLE FAMILY

From the age of about 15 months, when your little one can really start to tuck into family meals (albeit somewhat messily!), it makes things that little bit easier when preparing food for everyone. This applies to your go-to weekday meals, as well as dishes for more special occasions. In this chapter, I've provided some recipes that are particularly good for when you've got friends and family over. You want to prepare something suitable (and enjoyable!) for everyone – adults and little ones alike. Roast chicken (see page 269) always goes down well, in my experience, while slow-cooked pulled pork in a bun (see page 270) makes a fun meal for everyone to put together themselves. The Rainbow Veggie Tart (see page 267), meanwhile, not only looks impressive but also offers a crafty way of getting your kids to eat more veg!

This chapter also includes a range of healthy snacks for the whole family to enjoy and to keep hunger pangs at bay. The Kale Crisps, in a range of delicious flavours (see page 276), are super-easy to make and so much better for your little ones than a salt-laden bag of shop-bought crisps. Oatcake Fingers (see page 277) also make a great salt-free alternative to shop-bought ones. You could enjoy them spread with cream cheese, homemade nut butter (see page 280) or one of the dips in Chapter 5 (see pages 181 and 209). Muesli Cookies and On-The-Go Corn Muffins (see pages 279 and 274), both loaded with goodies, make the perfect portable snacks for when you're out and about with the family, helping to keep energy levels (and tempers!) on an even keel.

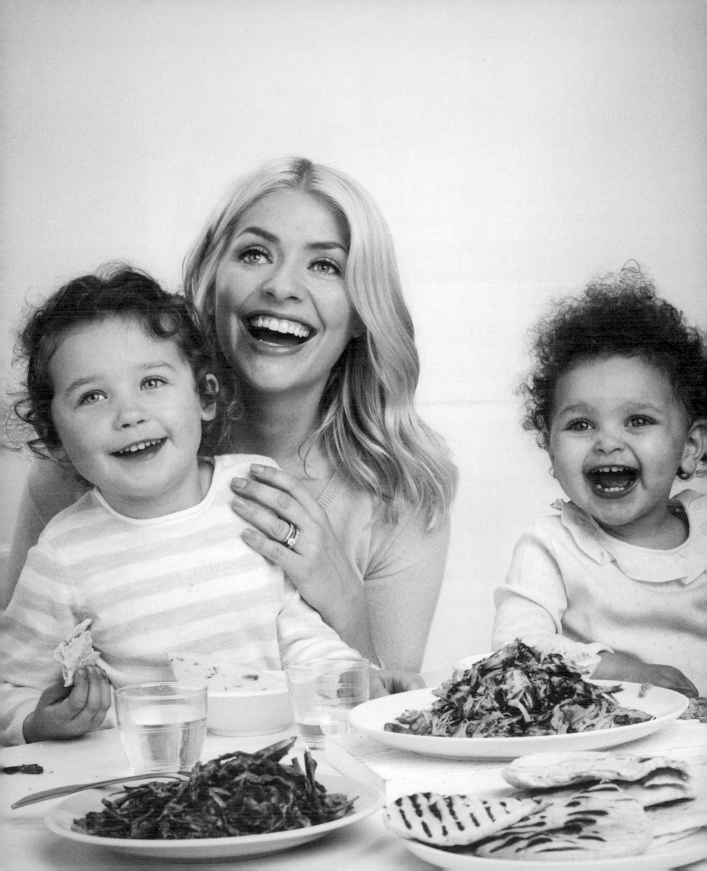

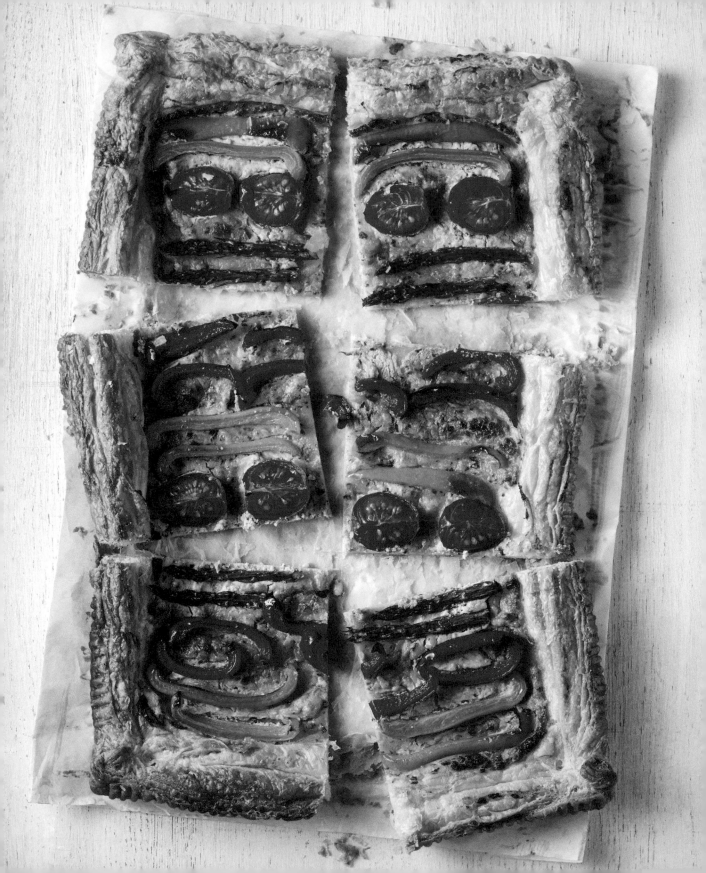

RAINBOW VEGGIE TART

Serves about 8

With its colourful topping of roasted vegetables, this puff pastry tart looks impressive and is a great way of encouraging kids to eat more veg. I've used yellow and red peppers, asparagus and tomatoes, but you can swap with your own favourites. Small broccoli or cauliflower florets, sliced courgette or red onion, or olives and a sprinkling of mozzarella or feta would all work well.

320g/11½oz ready-rolled puff pastry

1 egg, lightly beaten

75g/3oz full-fat cream cheese

3 tbsp basil pesto or Super-veg Green Pesto (see page 124)

1 small red pepper, deseeded and cut into 5cm/2in x 1cm/½in slices

1 small yellow pepper, deseeded and cut into 5cm/2in x 1cm/½in slices

8 small tomatoes, halved

16 asparagus tips, trimmed

1 tbsp olive oil, plus extra for brushing

1. Preheat the oven to 200°C/400°F/Gas 6.
2. Unroll the pastry and, keeping it on its greaseproof paper lining, lift it on to a baking tray. Brush the edge with a little of the beaten egg, then fold in the edges to make a 1cm/½in-wide border. Crimp the folded edges with the back of a fork.
3. Mix together the cream cheese and pesto, and spread the mixture over the pastry base in an even layer, avoiding the border.
4. Toss the red and yellow peppers, tomatoes and asparagus in the olive oil until coated, then arrange in rows on top of the cream-cheese mixture, starting with two rows of yellow pepper, a row of tomatoes, then two rows of asparagus and two rows of red pepper. Repeat, following the same sequence, until the pastry base is covered. Brush the top of the vegetables with a little extra oil, if needed.
5. Bake in the oven for 25 minutes or until the pastry is risen and golden – take a peek at the bottom to check it's cooked – and the vegetables are softened and starting to brown. Leave to cool slightly and cut into slices to serve.

SALMON PICNIC PIE

Serves 6–8 | ✱ *Suitable for freezing (pie only)*

A sort of posh giant 'sausage' roll! The flaky golden puff pastry comes with a salmon and creamy leek filling. It looks special enough to serve at a summery lunch for family and friends, or it can be eaten cold as part of a picnic. You could also make small individual pies, if you liked. Serve with a crisp mixed leaf salad.

2 leeks (about 350g/12oz total weight), finely chopped

2 tbsp crème fraîche

Finely grated zest of 1 unwaxed lemon

320g/11½oz ready-rolled puff pastry

700g/1½lb skinless, boneless salmon fillet of an even thickness, flesh patted dry

1 egg, lightly beaten

Freshly ground black pepper

For the lemon and chive yoghurt

125g/4½oz plain full-fat live yoghurt

1 tsp finely grated zest and juice of 1 unwaxed lemon

2 tbsp finely snipped chives

1. Preheat the oven to 220°C/425°F/Gas 7.
2. Steam the leeks for 3 minutes until just tender. Leave to cool slightly and then squeeze out the excess water – you want the leeks to be as dry as possible or they will make the pastry soggy. Put the leeks in a blender (or use a hand blender) with the crème fraîche and lemon zest, season with pepper and blend until just smooth.
3. Unroll the pastry, keeping it on its sheet of baking paper. Place the salmon fillet lengthways down one side of the pastry, about 2.5cm/1in from the edge. Spoon the leek mixture on top of the salmon.
4. Brush the long edge of the pastry nearest the filling with a little beaten egg, then fold the pastry over the top of the filling and press the two edges together. Trim any excess pastry and crimp the edge with the back of a fork or with your fingers. Lift the salmon roll on to a baking tray, using the baking paper to help you. Decorate the top of the roll with any leftover pastry, prick the top in a few places and brush with more beaten egg.
5. Bake in the oven for 40 minutes or until the pastry is crisp and golden, and the salmon is cooked through. While the pie is baking, mix together all the ingredients for the lemon and chive yoghurt. Remove the pie from the oven and leave to rest for 5 minutes or until ready to serve, then cut into slices and serve with the lemon and chive yoghurt and a mixed leaf salad.

ROAST CHICKEN WITH SMOKED PAPRIKA AND THYME STUFFING

Serves 4–6

I make no apologies for including a recipe for classic roast chicken. It makes the perfect family meal and is the ultimate comfort food. The smoked paprika, thyme and lemon stuffing keeps it moist while adding lots of flavour.

1.8kg/4lb chicken

50g/2oz unsalted butter, softened

50g/2oz fresh breadcrumbs

2 large garlic cloves, finely chopped

1 tbsp fresh thyme leaves

2 tsp mild smoked paprika

1 large unwaxed lemon

1 onion, cut into wedges

2 large carrots, scrubbed/peeled and cut into batons

Freshly ground black pepper

For the gravy

1 rounded tbsp plain flour

300ml/11fl oz low-salt chicken stock (for homemade Bone Broth, see page 111)

1. Take the chicken out of the fridge 1 hour before cooking. Preheat the oven to 190°C/375°F/Gas 5.
2. To make the stuffing, mix together two-thirds of the butter in a large bowl with the breadcrumbs, garlic, thyme and smoked paprika. Finely grate in the zest from the lemon then cut it in half.
3. Put the onion and carrots in a large roasting tin. Remove the string from the chicken and carefully loosen the skin on the breast. Push the stuffing mixture under the skin to cover the breast. Place the halved lemon inside the cavity, then sit the chicken on top of the veg. Smother the remaining butter over the outside of the chicken and season with pepper.
4. Roast the chicken in the oven for about 1½ hours, basting halfway through. To check it's cooked, pierce the thickest part of the thigh with a skewer – the juices should run clear and not pink.
5. Remove the chicken from the tin – as you lift it, pour any juices from the cavity into the tin. Cover the chicken with foil and leave to rest for 10–15 minutes.
6. To make the gravy, roughly mash the vegetables in the tin. Place it over a low heat, then stir in the flour and cook for a couple of minutes. Gradually pour in the stock, stirring and scraping off any sticky bits, then raise the heat and simmer for 2 minutes. Strain into a small pan, pressing the vegetables through the sieve, and simmer until thickened. Carve the chicken, adding any juices to the gravy before serving it.

SLOW-ROAST PIRI-PIRI PORK

Serves 8–10

Perfect for a summer gathering with friends and family, this slow-cooked pulled pork is best left to marinate overnight to get the full benefit of the smoky red-pepper marinade. Just before serving, place the pork, slaw, flatbreads or buns on separate plates or dishes on the table and let everyone help themselves.

1.5kg/3lb 4oz pork shoulder (skin on), scored

Olive oil, for rubbing into the pork

For the marinade

½ red pepper, deseeded and roughly chopped

1 small red onion, roughly chopped

2 large garlic cloves, chopped

1 tbsp olive oil, plus extra for brushing

2 tsp apple cider vinegar

1 tbsp mild smoked paprika

2 tsp dried oregano

4 tsp maple syrup

For the slaw

200g/7oz red cabbage, shredded

3 carrots, scrubbed/peeled and coarsely grated

1 raw beetroot, scrubbed and coarsely grated

225g/8oz plain full-fat live yoghurt

1. Mix together all the ingredients for the marinade, setting aside half of the maple syrup. Put the pork, skin-side down, on a rack in a dish and rub the marinade all over the meat side. Cover with cling film and leave to marinate in the fridge overnight.

2. Remove the pork 1 hour before roasting to let it come to room temperature and preheat the oven to 220°C/425°F/Gas 7.

3. Turn the pork over so the skin is facing upwards and pat it thoroughly dry with kitchen paper. Rub a little olive oil into the skin and place on the rack in a roasting tin. Roast in the oven for 20 minutes or until the skin starts to turn crisp and golden, then reduce the temperature to 150°C/300°F/Gas 2.

4. Remove the pork from the oven, pour a cupful of water into the bottom of the tin and cover the pork and tin with foil. Return the pork to the oven and cook for 4–5 hours or until it is incredibly tender. Remove the skin from the pork, cover the meat with foil and leave it to rest for 30 minutes.

5. If the skin needs crisping up, increase the oven temperature to 200°C/400°F/Gas 6 and return it to the oven to cook for another 15–25 minutes or until crisp and golden. Cut or break the crackling into pieces.

CONTINUES OVER THE PAGE

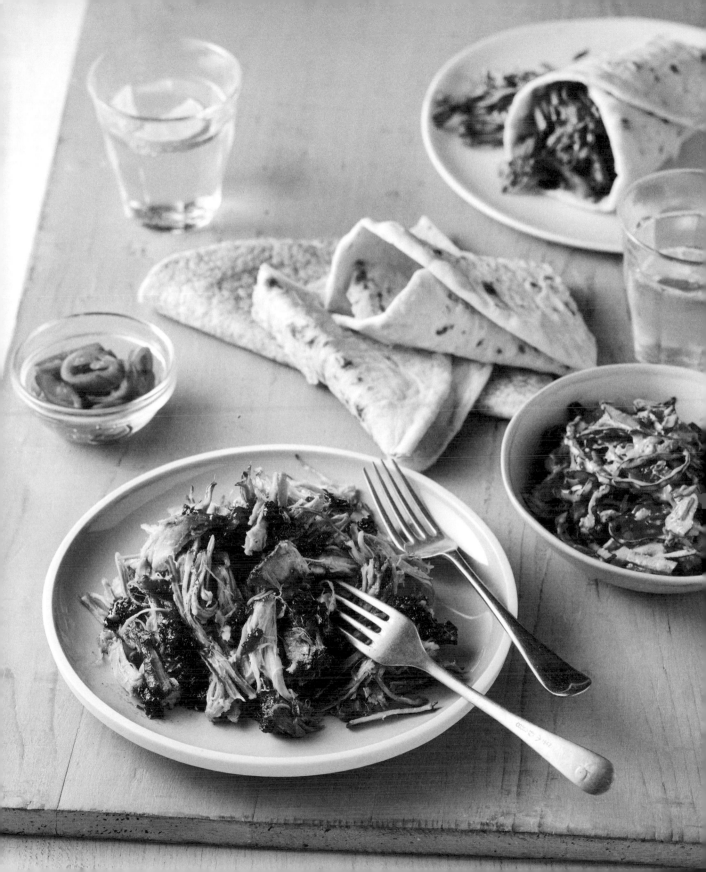

2 tsp wholegrain mustard

Juice of 1 lemon

To serve

Flatbreads, corn tortillas or brioche buns, warmed

Fresh jalapeño chillies, deseeded and sliced (optional)

6. To make the slaw, put the cabbage, carrots and beetroot in a serving bowl. Mix together the remaining ingredients to make a dressing, then pour it over the vegetables and turn until everything is mixed together.

7. For the piri-piri sauce, pour the roasting juices in the tin into a small saucepan, scoop off any fat from the top and stir in the saved maple syrup. Heat until the sauce has reduced and thickened slightly.

8. Using two forks, shred the meat and place on a serving plate with the crackling, spooning over as much of the sauce as needed. Serve the pork on warmed flatbreads or tortillas, or in a brioche bun, with a spoonful of slaw and with sliced jalapeño chillies for the grown-ups (if using).

BIG BEEF STEW WITH BAKED SWEET POTATOES

Serves about 8 | ❋ *Suitable for freezing*

The beauty of this stew is that it requires little attention while it cooks and all the preparation can be done a day or so in advance. Grown-ups may like to spice things up with a sprinkling of chilli flakes.

2–3 tbsp olive oil

1.25kg/2lb 12oz stewing steak, trimmed of fat and cut into 1.5cm/⅝in chunks

2 onions, chopped

200g/7oz butternut squash, peeled, deseeded and cut into bite-sized chunks

1 large red pepper, deseeded and chopped

3 garlic cloves, chopped

2 tsp ground cumin

1–2 tsp mild smoked paprika

1 tsp ground allspice

600ml/1 pint hot low-salt beef stock (for homemade Bone Broth, see page 110)

400g/14oz tin of green lentils

100g/3½oz cooked beetroot (not in vinegar), chopped

1 tsp dried chilli flakes (for the grown-ups – optional)

To serve

Sweet potatoes, scrubbed

Full-fat soured cream

1. Preheat the oven to 160°C/315°F/Gas 2½.
2. Heat half the olive oil in a large casserole dish, add half the beef and cook for 5 minutes over a medium-high heat or until browned all over. Scoop out using a slotted spoon and set aside. Brown the second batch of beef in the same way, adding a splash more oil, if needed, and set aside with the first batch.
3. Pour the rest of the oil into the casserole dish, add the onions and cook, covered, over a medium-low heat for 8 minutes or until softened, adding a splash of water if the pan is too dry. Add the squash, red pepper, garlic and spices, and cook, stirring, for a couple of minutes before returning the beef to the pan and pouring in the stock. Stir well and bring almost to boiling point, cover the pan and cook in the oven for 1½ hours.
4. Drain and rinse the lentils and put them in a jug with the beetroot. Blend until almost smooth using a hand blender, then add to the stew, stir well and replace the lid on the pan. At the same time put the sweet potatoes in the oven. Cook for another 1 hour or until the beef is tender (if the stew is too thick, add extra hot stock or water) and the sweet potatoes are cooked.
5. Serve with the baked sweet potatoes and a spoonful of soured cream. The grown-ups may like to stir some chilli flakes into their portion.

ON-THE-GO CORN MUFFINS

Makes 12 muffins | ❋ *Suitable for freezing*

These energizing corn muffins are easy to rustle up and make a change from the usual sandwich. Serve them plain or split in half and spread with soft cheese, guacamole (see page 249), hummus (see pages 197 and 201) or another favourite filling.

90g/3¼oz butter, melted, plus extra for greasing

140g/4¾oz plain flour

140g/4¾oz fine polenta

2 tsp baking powder

1 tbsp ground flaxseeds/linseeds

½ tsp sea salt

275g/10oz plain full-fat live yoghurt

100ml/3½fl oz full-fat milk

2 tsp lemon juice

2 eggs, lightly beaten

60g/2½oz mature Cheddar cheese, grated

Kernels from 1 large corn on the cob or 125g/4½oz tinned/frozen (and defrosted) sweetcorn, drained well and patted dry

3 spring onions, thinly sliced

½ small red pepper, deseeded and diced

You will need a 12-hole muffin tin and paper cases (optional)

1. Preheat the oven to 200°C/400°F/Gas 6 and liberally grease the muffin tin with butter or line with paper cases.
2. Mix together the flour, polenta, baking powder, flaxseeds and salt in a large bowl and make a well in the centre.
3. Whisk together the yoghurt, milk, lemon juice and eggs in a jug. Pour the yoghurt mixture into the dry ingredients and add the cheese, sweetcorn kernels, spring onions and red pepper. Using a wooden spoon, gently mix until everything is combined.
4. Spoon the batter into the prepared muffin tin and bake in the oven for 30–35 minutes or until risen and firm to the touch. Leave to sit in the tin for a few minutes before turning out on to a wire rack to cool.

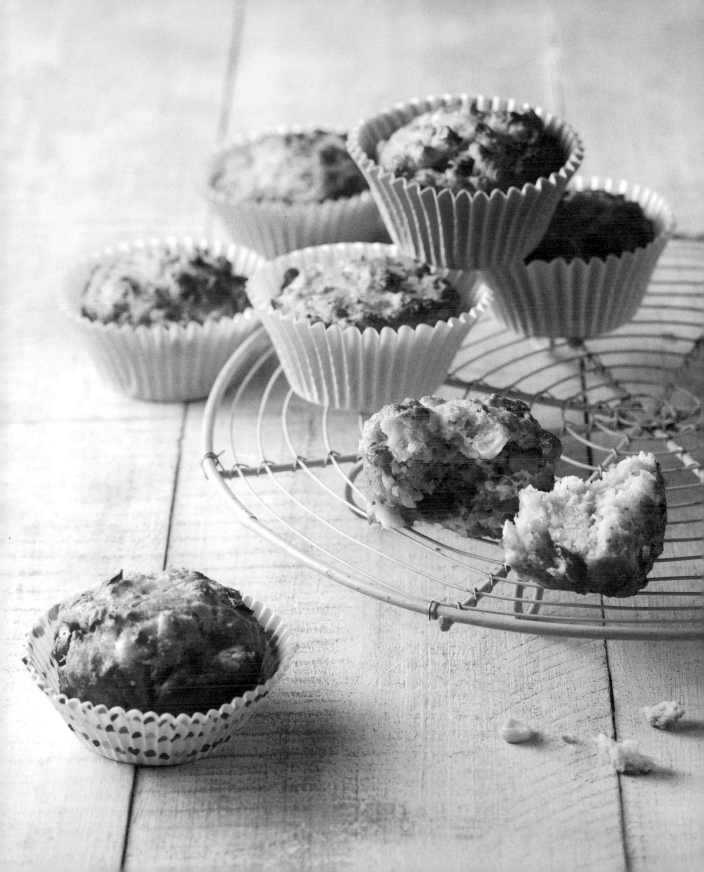

KALE CRISPS

Serves 4

Most children need a couple of nutrient-dense snacks a day to boost flagging energy and keep blood-sugar levels on an even keel. So, instead of grabbing a bag of crisps, why not try this baked crispy kale. I've suggested a few flavour options to ring the changes. The snack can also be crumbled up and sprinkled over rice and noodle dishes.

75g/3oz curly kale, tough stalks removed and leaves torn into bite-sized pieces

1 tsp cold-pressed rapeseed oil or coconut oil

1. Preheat the oven to 170°C/325°F/Gas 3.
2. Put the kale on a large baking tray, drizzle over the oil and then massage it into the leaves with your fingers until it gets into all the nooks and crannies. Spread the kale out in an even layer and bake in the oven for 15 minutes, turning once, until crisp. Keep a careful lookout as the kale cooks, as it can burn in a blink of an eye.
3. Remove from the oven and allow to cool. The kale crisps will keep stored in an airtight container for up to two days.

Flavour variations

* Smoky 'bacon': Mix ¾ teaspoon of mild smoked paprika into the rapeseed oil before drizzling over the kale leaves.
* Vegan 'cheese': Sprinkle 1 tablespoon of nutritional yeast flakes over the kale crisps after baking.
* Chinese 'seaweed': Replace the rapeseed oil with sesame oil and sprinkle ½ teaspoon of toasted sesame seeds, if you like, over the kale crisps after baking.
* Garlic: Sprinkle ½ teaspoon of garlic powder over the kale crisps after baking.

OATCAKE FINGERS

Makes 16 oatcakes

Find bags of oatmeal in the breakfast-cereal aisle in large supermarkets. Any leftovers can be used to make a lovely creamy porridge.

100g/3½oz medium oatmeal

175g/6oz wholemeal flour, plus extra for dusting

1 tbsp ground flaxseeds/ linseeds

1 tsp baking powder

Small pinch of salt

100g/3½oz unsalted butter, chilled, cut into small pieces

4 tbsp full-fat milk

1. Preheat the oven to 200°C/400°F/Gas 6 and line two baking sheets with baking paper.
2. Place the oatmeal, flour, ground flaxseeds, baking powder and salt in a large bowl and mix together.
3. Using your fingertips, lightly rub the butter into the flour mixture until it resembles fine breadcrumbs, then make a well in the centre. Pour in the milk and mix, first with a fork and then with your hands, to form a ball of dough.
4. Turn the dough out on a lightly floured work surface and knead briefly until smooth. Using a floured rolling pin, roll out the dough into a rectangle, about 5mm/¼in thick. Neaten the edges and cut the dough into 16 fingers.
5. Put the oatcake fingers on the prepared baking sheets and prick the top of each one three times with a fork. Bake in the oven for 15 minutes or until lightly golden, swapping the baking sheets around halfway through cooking. Leave to cool on a wire rack. You can store these in an airtight container for up to 5 days.

» Oats are loaded with beneficial vitamins, minerals and fibre, and can help improve blood-sugar control.

SNOWBALLS

Makes 15 balls

Pop a few of these energy-giving desiccated-coconut-coated balls into a lidded container and you're good to go. They're a perfect treat for keeping hungry tummies happy until mealtime. Choose unsulphured dark dried apricots rather than the bright orange ones, as not only do they come without preservatives but they taste really good, too.

100g/3½oz blanched hazelnuts

4 tbsp desiccated coconut, plus extra for coating

2 tbsp rolled porridge oats

100g/3½oz unsulphured dark dried apricots, chopped

3 tbsp fresh orange juice

Finely grated zest of ½ small unwaxed orange

1. Put the hazelnuts in a large, dry frying pan and toast over a medium-low heat, tossing the pan frequently, until they start to brown slightly and smell toasted. Remove from the heat and leave to cool.
2. Put the hazelnuts in a food processor and process until very finely chopped. Add the desiccated coconut and oats, and blitz briefly until partially chopped. Tip into a large bowl.
3. Place the apricots, orange juice and zest in a food processor and blitz to a thick paste, then stir into the hazelnut mixture.
4. Sprinkle enough desiccated coconut over a plate to cover. Shape the hazelnut mixture into 15 walnut-sized balls and roll them in the desiccated coconut until lightly coated. (You can also press the mixture, about 1cm/½in thick, into a large baking tray lined with baking paper and cut into fingers.) Store in an airtight container in the fridge for up to two weeks.

MUESLI COOKIES

Makes 16 cookies

Loaded with goodies and much lower in sugar than shop-bought biscuits, these simple cookies travel well if you're out and about. For an added treat, you could sandwich ice cream or frozen yoghurt between two cookies – they beat wafers hands down!

140g/4¾oz unsweetened muesli base (a mixture of grains, nuts and seeds)

50g/2oz ground almonds

40g/1½oz pecan nuts, roughly chopped

½ tsp ground cinnamon

1 ripe banana, peeled

1 tsp vanilla extract

2 tbsp maple syrup

4 tbsp coconut oil, melted

1. Preheat the oven to 180°C/350°F/Gas 4 and line two baking sheets with baking paper.
2. Place the muesli in a bowl with the ground almonds, pecans and cinnamon, and mix together. (If serving the cookies to young children, first blitz the muesli and pecan nuts in a food processor until very finely chopped.)
3. Using the back of a fork, mash the banana with the vanilla extract and maple syrup, and add to the bowl. Stir in the melted coconut oil and mix everything together until well combined.
4. Place heaped tablespoons of the mixture, spaced apart, on the prepared baking sheets, then flatten each one with your fingers into a thin round, about 5mm/¼in thick. The mixture should make about 16 cookies.
5. Bake in the oven for 20–25 minutes, swapping the baking sheets around halfway through cooking, until crisp and lightly golden. Leave on the trays for 5 minutes, then transfer the cookies to a wire rack to cool and crisp up further. You can store them in an airtight container for up to one week.

MIXED NUT BUTTER

Makes about 150g/5oz nut butter

Spread on rice cakes, bread, toast, oatcakes or slices of apple or pear, nut butter makes a quick, sustaining snack, while a spoonful added to a smoothie will help boost energy levels. Shop-bought peanut butter can be loaded with unwanted extras, such as palm oil, sugar and salt, but it's easy to make your own and you don't have to stick to just peanuts. This butter is a mixture of cashews – rich in zinc, iron and magnesium – and hazelnuts, which are especially high in copper, a mineral we need to keep our hair and skin healthy.

75g/3oz cashew nuts

75g/3oz blanched hazelnuts

2 tsp sunflower oil

1. Preheat the oven to 180°C/350°F/Gas 4.
2. Tip the cashews and hazelnuts on to a large baking tray and spread out evenly. Roast in the oven for 12 minutes, turning once, or until the nuts start to smell toasted and go brown.
3. Tip the nuts into a food processor and blitz until very finely chopped. Add the sunflower oil and continue to process the nuts until they turn into a smooth, thick paste. This takes a little time and patience, and you may need to occasionally scrape down the sides of the bowl to ensure the nuts are evenly blended. Depending on your processor, it will take about 10 minutes.
4. Once made, the mixed nut butter will keep for up to a week stored in a lidded jar in the fridge.

CHOC-NUT BUTTER

Makes about 125g/4½oz nut butter

Who could resist this healthier version of the popular shop-bought chocolate–nut spread? It uses Mixed Nut Butter (see page 280) as its base, but you could swap with a ready-made hazelnut butter instead (made with no added sugar or salt).

5 tbsp Mixed Nut Butter (see page 280)

1 tbsp coconut oil

1 tbsp honey or maple syrup

1 tbsp unsweetened cocoa or cacao powder

Beat together all the ingredients for the choc–nut butter. Store for up to a week in a lidded jar in the fridge.

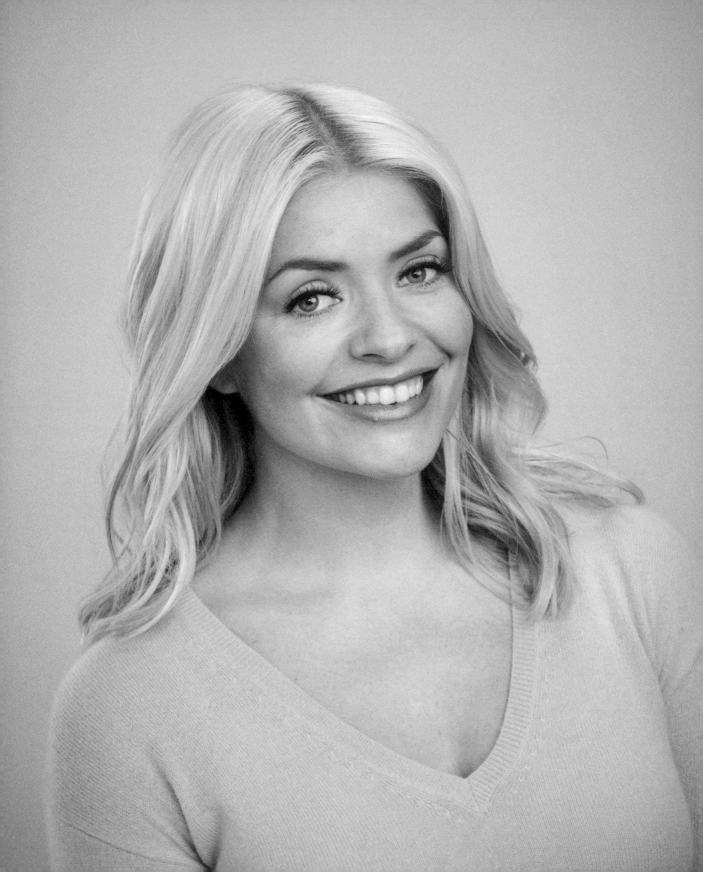

A FINAL WORD

Throughout this whole weaning journey, what you've got to remember is that all kids eventually learn to feed themselves. In fact, it won't be long before the words 'Mum, what can I have, I'm hungry' will be ringing in your ears for ever more! And when you're sitting there covered in splattered sweet potato and broccoli mush, thinking, Why won't this small person eat some food? Isn't he hungry? Am I not cooking properly? Doesn't my food taste nice? Don't forget, it's a big learning curve – for both of you. But you owe it to your child to set him off on the right track. And that's all about creating good eating habits, offering a range of healthy foods in a variety of flavours and textures. It's about giving him an education in table etiquette and in sharing a meal that will help him through life, enabling him to join in sociably with other people – including that all-important dinner date with a potential life partner! Sitting around the table isn't just about eating food. It's about fun and laughter, problems aired, stories shared, family getting together, Christmas dinner – all of those magical times.

Weaning is the start of a really exciting and important part of your baby's life. And it's not going to happen overnight. You will have realized by now that parenthood isn't about the quick fix. Nothing is immediate and babies develop at different rates. You've just got to take it slowly, listen to the needs of your baby and appreciate that what works one day might not work the next, but keep persevering and just take a deep breath and be patient. Patience is half the battle when it comes to weaning. You will get there and it will happen. And hopefully it will be fun along the way!

I think mealtimes should be an exciting, enjoyable time for you and your baby. While you're doing it, just keep asking yourself, 'What's my face doing at the moment? Does it look pained and stressed?' Remember that your baby takes in so much information from you and will absorb your emotional state. If you're pulling a face, or panicking or thinking, Just eat the food! with gritted teeth, your baby will pick up on that and feel anxious. You need to try to keep things really calm. Put some gentle music on. Sing. Make it fun. Play games. Maybe think back to your own childhood. My parents used to fly aeroplanes of food into my mouth, trains into the tunnel – anything to make it fun.

My favourite technique, which I tried with all of mine at different times, was to hold out a spoonful of food, close my eyes and say: 'Can you make it disappear, can you make it disappear? If I open my eyes and it's gone, you're magic!' And when they make it disappear, there's so much joy on their faces when you open your eyes, they actually feel like they have magic powers! That really works. Think of little tricks like this to get you through the tough times.

So, good luck and hang in there – it will happen!

ACKNOWLEDGEMENTS

First and foremost, I must say a huge thank you to my wonderful sister, Kelly. I'm so blessed to have so many supportive people in my life and none more so than she. Personally and professionally, she's always there to lend an ear, or a hand – particularly during those more testing parenting moments! Going through the weaning process four times with our little ones, we'd be constantly on the phone talking about what seemed to be working (and what didn't!). And now that I've come out the other side, I really wanted to share our varied experiences with you and pass on all the useful things we've learnt along the way. But for me to put my thoughts out there in the form of a book, I need someone who can unlock my mind and transform my thoughts into words on the page. Luckily for me, writing is Kelly's passion and her gift, and so Truly Scrumptious Baby was born.

My next big thank you goes to my parents. Mum and Dad – all the strong values I try and instil in my own family are the ones that you instilled in us. I treasure my childhood memories of mealtimes. We were so lucky to spend so much time together at the dinner table, and it was only when I became a parent myself that I realised how tricky that can be! So much of my approach to cooking and feeding the family has come from you both – from the meals we had as children to the importance of family being together around the table.

To Dan, Harry, Belle and Chester – thank you for being the best family I could ever have hoped for. I feel truly blessed to have you in my life. One of my favourite places to be is sat together around our kitchen table; watching you eat, share stories and laugh. Those moments are actually a real gauge of how much you've all grown and it fills my heart with joy to know that, no matter what changes come, mealtimes will always be a constant in our family - the place where we come together to regroup and connect. Daniel, thank you for being the best dinner quiz master ever!!! Whilst putting this book together, I've been flooded with

so many beautiful memories, from those first spoonfuls of baby rice to demolishing birthday cakes! You're the inspiration for this book and all the recipes and guidance in it, so thank you.

There are loads of people who have been instrumental in getting this book off the ground. Particular thanks have to go to my editor at HarperCollins, Zoe, who's worked tirelessly with Kelly and me to replicate the exact book I saw in my mind – which is no mean feat! Massive thanks, also, to the rest of the publishing team – James, George, Isabel and Katie in particular.

I also want to say an extra special thank you to Emily at James Grant Management, who goes above and beyond for me every single day… Emily, you are amazing! And thank you also to Rowan, Rachel, and the rest of the James Grant team for your unwavering dedication and support.

And I must, of course, say a huge thank you to all the Truly Scrumptious Babies (and your wonderful parents!) for allowing us to take so many gorgeous photos of you for the book. To Darcy, Elsie, George, Rudy, Grace and Amarrio – you were all consummate professionals and I loved every single one of my cuddles! To the rest of the shoot team, too, thank you so much for working so hard to capture the most beautiful images. To Danielle Wood, Fern Green and Lydia Brun, who produced the most scrumptious food photography, and to Jay Brooks, Lauren Miller, Angie Smith, Ciler Pekash and Patsy O'Neill for all your hard work.

And finally, thanks to each and every one of you who picks up this book and trusts me to help guide you through such an important step in your baby's life. Weaning is undoubtedly stressful at times but it's also one of the most wonderful experiences you'll have, and the satisfaction of seeing your little one's face light up when they try something that piques their taste buds makes it all worthwhile, I promise!

Love, Holly xxx

A FINAL WORD

INDEX